Contents

Exercises

Notice to Readers

Laws are constantly changing. Every effort is made to keep this publication as current as possible. However, the author, the publisher, and the vendor of this book make no representations or warranties regarding the outcome or the use to which the information in this book is put and are not assuming any liability for any claims, losses, or damages arising out of the use of this book. The reader should not rely on the author or the publisher of this book for any professional advice. Please be sure that you have the most recent edition.

The information presented in this book is not intended as medical advice or as a substitute for medical counselling. The information should be used in conjunction with the guidance and care of your physician. Consult your physician before implementing any exercise program or movement changes you feel could be harmful to your health. Obtain the consent of your physician and/or work with your physician throughout the duration of your time using the recommendations in this book, as you are agreeing to accept full responsibility for your actions.

Dedication

For my wife, Le Le, who moves me every day.

"Knowing is not enough, we must apply.
Willing is not enough, we must do."

— Bruce Lee

Introduction:
The Power of Movement

At some point, all of us have struggled to maintain our health whether trying to stay fit, recovering from illness, avoiding illness, or taking care of our mental health. *Move or Die* focuses on time spent sitting, not as a problem to eradicate, but as an opportunity: Start moving, and you can lead a healthier and happier life.

By judo-flipping our sedentary time, we can transform sitting time into an opportunity to enhance our health in ways that were not possible before. With a healthier workforce, organizations and companies experience more productivity and by extension, profit. The most difficult part is changing your mindset. After that, all you need to do is move.

This book is your guide to rethinking popular approaches to health, then opening the door to a new world of movement, different from traditional forms of exercise. It shows you how to incorporate movement throughout your day, elevating your energy, mood, and health.

By now, you may have heard that sitting is the new smoking. A large and growing body of research connects prolonged sitting and sedentary behavior with serious health problems like cancer, diabetes, obesity, and more. However, prolonged sitting doesn't only impact our physical health. The more we sit the more other aspects of us become rigid, like behavior, thinking, communication, and relationship patterns. The problem of being sedentary is a symptom of a larger problem: a generalized stagnation resulting in the stiffening of bodies, the fixation of minds, the staleness of relationships, and the eventual disruption of growth throughout entire organizations.

This book introduces movement as a mindset. It will help you develop the skills to become aware of unhealthy patterns and help you explore choices to move towards healthier possibilities that allow for growth. Central to this work is the creation and pursuit of freedom of movement. Freedom is at the heart of many of our deepest values: freedom of choice, freedom to love whom we wish, financial freedom, freedom of speech, freedom of religion, and the freedom to vote. We have yet to prioritize our bodies and movement in the same way, particularly in our working environments.

The freedom to move our bodies is central to experiences of optimal health. Movement is the key to accessing resources, creativity, and innovation that can otherwise be trapped when our bodies and our minds are locked in a sitting position for hours on end. When I am discussing movement, I am not just talking about physical movement but also psychological, relational, and organizational.

The relationship between physical health and other aspects of our lives should be obvious. We exist within bodies so it makes sense that if our bodies are stuck, other areas of our lives get stuck as well. Sitting down for long periods reduces blood flow and the production of hormones and neurochemicals. This has an impact on our mental health.

My hope is to inspire you to incorporate the power of movement into your day so you can transform your mind, body, relationships, and organizations by adding new energy, new perspectives, new strength, and an authentic experience of health. I will help you do this by teaching a philosophy of health called the Freedom of Movement. Life is a complex process that requires constant learning and growing: the freedom to move one's mind, body, and relationships is an important method for coping with challenges and facilitating growth.

1. The Philosophy of the Freedom of Movement

The power of movement is found in the freedom it can create for people who use and integrate it into their lives. I have discovered the freedom of movement in my own life. It has been a force that has given me more health, energy, and a deeper connection to myself. Here are a few of the lessons that will be elaborated upon throughout this book:

- There is no one right way to move. Be fluid and willing to experiment and explore until you find a way to incorporate movement that fits you and your life.

- There is always a choice as it relates to your health and body. People do not function in a healthy way when things are forced or when there are rigid rules of what they should or have to do. Having to sit still is one of those rigid rules that needs to be transformed and made into a choice instead of a mandate.

- Take responsibility for your health. No person, tool, gadget, or program can help move your body for you. Each individual needs to take responsibility to move. No one can be moved.

- Have no set patterns. Focus on keeping Freedom of Movement in all areas of your life. Avoid patterns which create stagnation. Create new moves every day as well as new thoughts, new relationships, and new methodologies. Keep things fresh. Keep focused on your purpose, which is your mission and vision, and update as needed.

- Your body is a part of nature so it contains a wealth of resources and wisdom. It is naturally oriented to move towards growth and healing. Simply learning to listen to its needs and responding appropriately is a large step towards health.

- Different domains of health interact dynamically so changes in one realm can lead to changes in the others, whether intended or not. For example, freeing the body can also free one's thinking.

This book helps you transform your sedentary time into an opportunity to improve your health through information, techniques, and skills that will empower you to incorporate movement throughout your day. While the practices are simple and usually only take a minute at a time, they challenge old beliefs and patterns. By learning the power of movement and the freedom it can provide, you will have more control of your mind, your choices and, most importantly, your health.

2. The Problem of Sitting Is a Problem of Not Listening to the Body

According to the Center for Disease Control and Prevention (CDC), chronic diseases and conditions such as heart disease, stroke, cancer, diabetes, obesity, and arthritis are among the most common, costly, and preventable of all health problems. Research has shown significant connections between prolonged sitting and many chronic illnesses.

Beyond sitting, I believe that the source of these health problems begins when people disconnect themselves from their bodies. The position of sitting and the problem of being sedentary exemplifies this pattern of ignoring the body. The longer we sit hunched over keyboards facing screens without movement, the more unfamiliar we become with our bodies, their signals and needs. This internal pattern of being disconnected and not listening to our bodies can become a relationship pattern when individuals stop communicating their needs to their colleagues and managers within an organization or any system.

This dynamic of not listening to one's body perpetuates poor self-care because people begin to disconnect and distrust themselves and their environment. People with this kind of closed behavior become silent not only on matters that impact them personally like their health, but also on issues that directly impact the health of any business with which they are involved.

Without the ability to listen to our bodies and the ability to communicate openly with others, problems and concerns both personal and professional remain hidden until it is too late and employees experience burnout and need to take stress leave. Some companies try to incorporate health and wellness programs, but it is not yet well understood how health practices can be incorporated into the flow of daily work. The approaches are often singular, as they focus on the body separate from the activities of work. For example, offering gym memberships, or installing a gym in the space, or bringing in a yoga instructor. The body and health are still addressed in isolation from the rest of what is happening in the workplace. A healthy body, primarily through working out and going to the gym, becomes another pressure-filled task amongst an ever growing to-do list. It often falls to the bottom of that list instead of being integrated naturally into the flow of daily activities happening in the workplace.

The ThinkMOVE approach invites people to integrate the needs of their bodies throughout their workdays. This is done by emphasizing movement, not exercise, and incorporating many short breaks of movement throughout the day to offset sedentary time. This approach enhances the individual's health and their ability to work productively by adding focus and energy to the work day. By teaching self awareness, in particular body awareness skills, the ThinkMOVE program encourages motivated and self-directed movement breaks. By listening to what is happening in the body and periodically asking what it needs, it is a short distance to resolving those needs. For example, instead of ignoring a sore back which could eventually become a herniated disc, an individual can choose to stand up and stretch for a minute every half hour to relieve the tension.

We can also make changes to our environment that can help. One simple change is to create spaces where people have the freedom to take whatever physical position (standing, sitting, moving, etc.), they want during the workday, and give them the freedom to change positions whenever needed. Freedom of Movement will help people take care of their bodies and express their individuality. This creates an organizational culture where people feel more empowered, autonomous, and relaxed.

One can imagine a group or company that practices this will be more likely to freely express their creative ideas as well as concerns about problematic processes happening in the company, compared to a group of sedentary office workers who strain their bodies to sit for ten or more hours a day, ignoring signals and never communicating needs because they do not feel safe or welcome to do so. Participants in the ThinkMOVE program report experiencing greater engagement with colleagues and across their company hierarchy. Research also demonstrates the relationship between exercise and creative thinking.

Companies that are not investing in their employees' health don't see how healthy bodies lead to healthy minds which relate to healthy relationships, and how taken together these connections positively impact the health and growth of a business. Each of these areas consists of various skills that make employees more competent including self/ body awareness, communication skills, and clarity and commitment to the larger purposes and vision of the organization. Without all of these elements functioning in a healthy way, toxic and maladaptive patterns begin to develop within individual employees and between employees that can negatively impact the organization as a whole.

Imagine that Kevin, a 32-year-old computer programmer who is sedentary, overweight, and depressed, is working long hours, and is hardly able to keep up with his work. He can't find time to go the gym, let alone eat a healthy lunch. Unhealthy work processes persist for Kevin because there are organizational rules against commenting on the situation or complaining. There are unspoken rules in this company that good employees make sacrifices, work hard, work long hours, and never complain. The hardest working employees are perceived as those sitting at their desks continuously without needing breaks. Kevin placates to his manager by accepting new projects without hesitation. He never voices or asserts his own needs or limitations as they relate to his body or mind. This situation continues to deteriorate as the quality of Kevin's health declines along with the quality and efficiency of his work. The lack of freedom to comment or even move could be the beginning steps towards the degradation of the company as many employees share Kevin's experience and talk about it in closed quarters. Morale lowers and the company's resilience and agility is lost.

The necessary paradigm shift is a transformation of perception; one that sees health not as a component that is separate from work but as the resource that makes work possible. The health of individuals, relationships, and the organization are all interconnected. Health as it relates to these different areas is just as, if not more, important than money. Money is an important indicator of the financial health of the organization just as blood pressure is an indicator of heart health, but health of the employees is truly the lifeblood of any company.

This book aims to guide individuals and companies towards listening and communicating honestly with themselves and each other so everyone feels respected and valued. In safety and acceptance, people become more open to communicating and sharing their needs. This requires a transformation in the way we think about the workplace.

3. Moving from a Workplace to a Lifeplace

"Work," "workplaces," "working out," being a "workaholic." All of this emphasis on work reminds me of the Greek myth of Sisyphus pushing a rock up a hill only to have it roll back down for eternity. Work without a meaningful purpose quickly turns into drudgery. I have never met anyone who works for work's sake; although I have seen many people stuck in this mindset. They have expectations about what work should be. That it should hurt or else it isn't really working. That it should be endured. That it shouldn't be fun or joyful.

When it comes to work, there is always a deeper purpose connected to life. Even working at jobs we aren't passionate about, we are providing for ourselves and our families in order to live. We are making a living. When we focus just on work and the workplace, we lose sight of a larger vision of life and how our daily activities are connected. In our devotion to work, we stop listening to our bodies. This becomes the source of many health problems. A singular focus on work squeezes out the possibility of health.

I am not a fan of work. I don't like putting the frame of "work" around all my daily activities; particularly the activities where I spend most of my time. To me, there is no life in that. Work or working hard becomes a barrier to life instead of being a part of life. For a long time, people have been trying to create work/life balance, but to balance one thing against another means they are distinct and separate.

The concept of 9:00 a.m. to 5:00 p.m. being for work and the rest of our life (family, hobbies, rest, exercise) needing to fall outside of this timeframe seems to be a recipe for disease. This artificial separation makes work so unappealing that I believe this is a major reason why a majority of people are unhappy at their jobs.

I no longer think about transitioning from work to life or from life to work. To me, there is no need for work/life balance because it is all life. I focus and do what needs to be done. Everything I do is all serving the same purpose: to live life to the fullest by helping to move the world. This way I don't spend time on things that are not supportive to my life or that are unacceptable to me. I simply do what I feel expands life as it relates to my vision and values and that is all.

Take a moment to reflect on why your company or the company you work for exists. Hopefully it is because it provides a product or service that makes life better for other people, the community or the environment. Hopefully this purpose fits with your goals and values and hopefully you are paid a living wage that enables you to take care of yourself and your family. This is all in service of life, not work.

Take a moment to reflect on the word "work." What associations does it conjure?

Some of the words that come up for me include: hard, chores, boring, painful, endless, tiring, not fun, disciplined, sweat, turmoil. I want to be clear: I'm not saying that there isn't a place for work or that these associations are inherently bad, but simply that negative experiences shouldn't be central. So what's the alternative?

What I propose is that we transform our workplaces into Lifeplaces. If we focus on how our activities create and improve life instead of just thinking about it as work, how much more of ourselves would we be willing to bring to this Lifeplace? Hard work is just one resource of many that belong in the Lifeplace. Other resources that people could bring could be creativity, commitment, intelligence, joy, and passion. How much more joy and commitment could people have for what they are doing if they could honestly tell themselves that they aren't just going to work to work hard, but that they are moving towards and creating life?

Most employers would be happy to have employees who could bring such a rich version of themselves to serve their customers or clients. This is another way of describing employee engagement: Specifically that employees are free to show up as whole people, not just a compartmentalized workaholic version of themselves.

Personally, I am more than willing to work hard, to cry, and to bleed, if it brings something meaningful and positive into the world. I also want to bring my joy, commitment, creativity, fun, and love to that creation. This is the vision I have for healthy organizations. Making the choice to freely move our bodies and our minds makes so many more resources available to us that can be used to serve the mission, vision, and purpose of our Lifeplaces.

Taking a step back to reframe the language around work and focusing on life opens up new possibilities and invites new conversations. Instead of asking "What do you do for work?" we might begin to ask (ourselves first, then each other), "What do you do to create life or to connect to life?" or "What do you do to make life better for others?" or "What do you do that gives you the feeling of life or of being alive?" Calling it a Lifeplace creates space to include our physical, mental, and relationship health, alongside creating products and services that help make life better for others.

> The master in the art of living makes little distinction between his work and his play, his labor and his leisure, his mind and his body, his education and his recreation, his love and his religion. He hardly knows which is which. He simply pursues his vision of excellence at whatever he does, leaving others to decide whether he is working or playing. To him he is always doing both.

> — James A. Michener

As we have been discussing, there are several broad categories of health which we might further describe as psychological, physical, social, and organizational. Trying to address each of these areas separately is analogous to the story of the four blind men and the elephant. The story goes that there are four blind men trying to determine what the elephant is by feeling different parts of the animal. One of the blind men feels a leg and says the elephant is like a pillar. The one who feels the tail says the elephant is like a rope. The one who feels the tusks says the elephant is a solid pipe. The one feels the belly says the elephant is a like a wall. Each man is correct in his own way; however, they are each merely describing features of a greater whole.

Compartmentalization and alienation between the domains of health creates conflict and misses the whole picture. Often trainings, interventions, and programs focus on one domain to the exclusion of others. Some examples include mental health services offered by an employer to see a psychotherapist off-site; teambuilding workshops to improve relationships and communication within a team; gym memberships or onsite Yoga classes for physical health; and retreats or conferences for leadership training with visioning exercises for organizational health. Trying to improve health in these four domains separately from each other is like trying to drive a car with the wheels, engine, seats, and frame all disconnected.

4. Movement Education

In order to move, education is the key; not just in terms of physical aspects of health, but health in all domains.

The lines we create that separate areas of health are useful. They give us a focus and concrete plans and practices for each domain. By exploring the spaces between these different categories of health we can learn about their interactions and the positive impacts of improving all domains simultaneously. This focus on the relationship between categories can invite new questions: "How does my mindset impact my relationships and the organization?" "How will paying attention to my body's needs improve my health?" "How can greater individual health improve the quality of work the organization produces?"

By learning to apply the Freedom of Movement philosophy, the approach is not to try to address each category separately, but to integrate them by applying general principles and mindsets that are health- and growth-oriented. Certain principles flow from a state of health, whether you are talking about physical, mental, relationship, or organizational health. Some of these are awareness, nurturance, integration, fluidity, openness, honesty, balance, attunement, listening, and congruence.

To make significant and sustainable change, we need to explore the interplay of the four domains of health. This will result in healthier people, relationships, and organizations which, from business perspective, create a foundation for financial growth for companies as well.

The artificial separation of the four domains of health is a large part of the problem we face when it comes to health and also job dissatisfaction. This separation represents a way of living (or *not* living) that creates and perpetuates rigid patterns of being. Being sedentary epitomizes this separation. During long periods of sitting, the body's needs and sensations are removed from conscious awareness for the sake of work. To fit into the workplace one learns to restrict oneself to a specific series of movements which consist of sitting, with only a few trips perhaps to the photocopier or washroom.

Being sedentary is a pattern we develop that impacts the body, the mind, relationships, and organizations as a whole. All of these domains overlap and create a cascade effect that can either accumulate health or disease. Organizational health is particularly significant because it doesn't just overlap with the other domains, it encapsulates them. The other elements exists within that context.

Consider an example of integrating the skills of body awareness, movement and communication and its impact at the organizational level.

Sally is feeling tired, disconnected, and stuck on a project. She takes a moment to become aware of her body and asks herself how her body is feeling right then. She realizes she feels stiff from sitting for several hours. She also recognizes her accumulating stress from feeling stuck in her work. She decides to get up and connect with her colleague, Maria, through a MOVE break. They connect through movement doing some light stretches. Sally talks about something she's stuck on, and asks directly for help. She first asks if Maria would be willing to help and puts out an invitation without demanding it. Sally practices communication and healthy boundaries, which means she is direct and open with her needs and also open to Maria's needs and limits. Maria has the option and opportunity to practice saying a real yes or no to being helpful. By tuning in and listening to her whole body, Maria can be aware of whether she is able to take on another project or not. Fortunately, she is. Sally walks away from the interaction feeling supported by her colleague, confident that she is not alone and is moving in a good direction, as well as refreshed and energized by the movement.

Movement occurred in terms of physical movement but also in Sally's willingness to move her mind as she decided to listen to her body. She also moved her relationship with Maria by her willingness to communicate her needs and ask for help. These movements of minds, bodies, and relationships help create a healthy flow within the organization.

> *If you don't understand and appreciate human movement, you won't really understand yourself or play. Learning about self-movement creates a structure for an individual's knowledge of the world; it is a way of knowing. Through movement play, we think in motion. Movement structures our knowledge of the world, space, and time so completely that we need to take a step back (a movement metaphor) to realize how much we think in these terms. Our knowledge of the physical world, based in movement, explains why we describe emotions with terms like "close," "distant," "open," "closed."*
>
> *We say we "grasp" an idea or "wrestle" with them, or "stumble" upon them. Movement play lights up the brain and fosters learning, innovation, flexibility, adaptability and resilience. These central aspects of human nature require movement to be fully realized.*
>
> — Dr. Stuart Brown, Psychiatrist and Researcher of Play and author of the book *Playing*

5. How This Book Works

In this book, you will find everything you need to start your own MOVE program in your life or at your office including the specific techniques needed to incorporate movement breaks as well as specific exercises that will help improve your body awareness, cardio, strength, core/balance, and flexibility. By incorporating movement throughout your day you will be addressing many of the health issues caused by a sedentary lifestyle, but more importantly you will develop an awareness of yourself that is inherently rewarding and healthy. With the information and tools in this book, you will create a deeper connection to yourself by acting in ways that are caring and loving towards your body.

In the first chapter, we focus on making the mindset shift necessary to begin to incorporate movement at the workplace. I will share the story of how the ThinkMOVE program was created. Hopefully some of my struggles and insights will resonate with you and save you some of the pain I had to experience before I created the ThinkMOVE approach.

In Chapter 2, we explore how a focus on movement and health makes business sense. Movement will not only prevent healthcare costs from rising, it will also increase productivity and connections within the office. This chapter on the business case for movement will be valuable to anyone in need of a coherent and cogent presentation of facts and logic to convince an organization to invest in health and wellness.

In Chapter 3, we look at the importance of shifting our culture and mindset to adapt new ways of working; specifically, ways that account for our health. Chapter 4 reviews the research that informs the program and gives you the key principles that help you incorporate movement into your day. Chapter 5 shows a model of change which is relevant to health, relationships, or organizational changes. This section will prepare you for what you and your company will experience along your moving journey. In Chapter 6, we offer an overview of the program.

In Chapter 7, I offer a specific definition of health as a renewable resource that enables us to achieve meaningful goals. This will help you prioritize your health by seeing how it is connected to everything you do. I have also included a Health Resource Self-Assessment (HRSA) in Chapter 8 that will help you become aware of your health resources and how you currently use them. Finally, in Chapter 9, we conclude with reflections on the benefits of incorporating these principles and values of movement in our everyday lives.

On the download kit, you will find all the exercises from this book as well as my sources and places to look for further reading.

Here are suggestions to help you get the most out of this book.

1. **Do:** Do the exercises throughout the book. You will not only move more and feel healthier, you'll also learn the underlying principles for incorporating any healthy behavior you wish.

2. **Share:** Sharing is caring for yourself and your friends. Find at least one other person who will take this movement journey with you. By helping others, you will help transform the culture of your workplace so that it is happier and healthier.

3. **Feel:** The program is an embodied practice so it will only work if you do the practices and let yourself move and feel what you feel. You will learn to listen to your whole body and develop a deeper connection with yourself through this awareness.

1

ThinkMOVE: An Origin Story (and How to Begin)

1. How Did ThinkMOVE Come to Be?

The development of my program to combat the sedentary lifestyle is so intimately connected to my life and my own pain that it often feels like destiny. It is perhaps no small coincidence that my last name is Sitt.

When I was 15 I looked like I do in Figure 1.

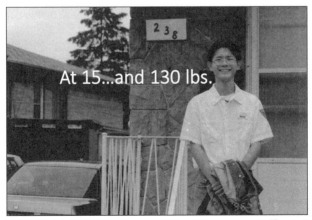

Figure 1

I was 130 lbs. and I hated being called skinny. One of my friends called me "Pie Gwut!" which means pork ribs in Chinese. At the time, I connected being skinny with being weak. After reading Arnold Schwarzenegger's biography, I was inspired to pack on some muscle. At this time, I made two decisions: I wanted to become a therapist so I could help other 15-year-olds navigate this angst-ridden, confusing, heart wrenching time, and I wanted to look like Arnold Schwarzenegger.

Ten years, and many chicken breasts later I competed in a body-building competition and looked like I do in Figure 2.

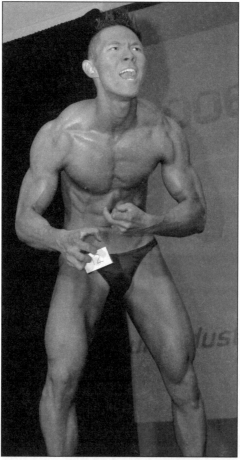

Figure 2

From this experience, I gained a sense of mastery over my body. I felt strong and capable; the feelings I had been yearning for. I learned how to train and eat healthfully to shape my body to look a certain way and I had the confidence and desire to help others to do the same.

Bodybuilding seemed a way of expressing ideal health. Exercise, or so I thought, was a way of reaching my greatest physical potential.

Inspired by my experience with bodybuilding, I became a personal trainer while I was in graduate school studying to become a therapist. I had a vision of one day bringing mental and physical health together. I had bought into and become a proponent of traditional methods of health and fitness. At that time, I knew little of the corporate world and how life as a desk jockey impacted people's health.

I thought I was healthy because I looked healthy and because I exercised and ate healthy foods. I didn't realize that as a personal trainer/graduate student I also had the benefit of never being in an office, glued to a chair for ten hours a day. I was running from class to class, on my feet, training clients, constantly shifting from my house, to the library, and school. I was moving all the time.

After graduating from the University of Toronto with a Master of Social Work degree, I started my first office job as a child and family therapist. Just like the first day of school, I was shown my little space with a desk and a chair with the presumption that "this is how you will work best: with your butt in this chair. All day." At the time, I had no reason to question this way of living/working since I had learned so well from many years of school to sit still, be quiet, and not to move or fidget. Little did I realize how hazardous to my health this would be.

After three years of working in an office and driving in rush hour traffic two hours a day, I went from weighing 165 pounds as a personal trainer to weighing close to 200 lbs as an office worker (see Figure 3).

I was burnt out, overweight, and depressed. I thought my weight gain was a result of aging and a slowing metabolism since I had continued to eat and exercise the same way I had as a graduate student.

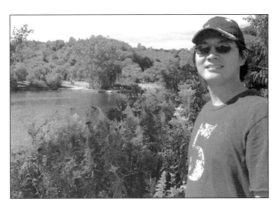

Figure 3

By January 2012, I had found a new job much closer to home. I was thrilled to cut down my commute from a few hours to only 15 minutes! On my second day at my new job, a snowstorm covered the city in ice and snow. Everything was beautifully white, like a blank page. The perfect image for a fresh start.

On my way home that evening I was walking through a parking lot, and there was an area that I suspected was covered in black ice. I approached with extreme caution, almost tiptoeing, like I was sneaking up on someone, but you can probably guess what happened next.

I fell hard. One of those falls that if you ever saw someone else do it you'd probably laugh heartily and maybe feel bad later: feet in the air, butt crashing onto the snow-covered concrete. BOOM! There I was lying on the ground thinking, "Help! I've fallen and I really can't get up!"

Snow landed on my face, and I was completely helpless. My back was wrecked. The pain was searing and shooting through my entire body. Eventually I managed to limp home and laid on my living room floor with ice packs.

The next morning, I visited a chiropractor. The doctor was very kind and after she did an assessment of my body she surprised me by asking, "Do you have to sit down a lot for your job?"

I nodded.

"How many hours would you say you sit a day?"

I gave it some thought: I sit during breakfast, then in my car, then at the office writing reports, seeing clients, meetings, lunch, then home in the car, then dinner, then I'm in front of the TV or computer in the living room for the rest of the evening. I sit all the time, I realized as I said, "Around 12 to 13 hours a day."

"Uh-hmm," she said knowingly. Then she said something that forever changed the way I think about health.

"Tim, falling was definitely not good for your back, but the real problem is you sit all day. Your body is incredibly stiff. You are tight throughout your hips, hamstrings, glutes, and quads. Sitting makes you inflexible like a dried elastic band ready to crack and therefore you were more prone to injury."

"But I work out," I protested.

"Doesn't matter. One hour of exercise isn't going to reverse what you do for 12 hours a day." She was telling me that what I knew about being healthy was incomplete. I had no idea how to fix the problem.

She handed me a paper with exercises and explained that I was to do them every one to two hours throughout my day to rehabilitate my back and disrupt sedentary time.

My first reaction was, "Ugh! Work? You're the doctor, can't you just fix me with an adjustment? Why do I have to do these weird exercises in the middle of my office multiple times a day? I'm busy with work. I have clients to see, phone calls to make, tons of paperwork, and meetings. I don't have time for this!" But I smiled at her politely, knowing that even though I wanted to get better I had no intention of doing my exercises. I held the attitude that the onus of care was on the healthcare professional.

At the time, I didn't realize how disempowering this relationship between professional and patient was, but now I see it as a "fix me" dynamic that pervades many of our interactions with doctors, physiotherapists, psychotherapists, and even our relationships with technologies such as wearables, apps, and any of the latest fitness equipment. Looking back, I also realize the attitude underlying my reaction was "I don't have time for my health during the workday." So I neglected it. I just couldn't imagine myself doing exercises at the office. There seemed to be too many barriers: How would I remember to do them? How often was I to do them? Where could I do them? What if someone saw me exercising at work? The practical considerations seemed to be outweighed by the looming sense of shame and embarrassment I would feel if I was caught moving my body at work.

A month went by and although the acute pain was gone, a dull ache and chronic feeling of vulnerability remained. I was seeing the chiropractor twice a week but I was still not doing my daily rehab exercises and I was not getting better.

I lived in constant fear of re-injuring my back. I was afraid of lifting weights, playing sports, and even simple actions like getting in and out of my car. I hated the feeling that I could not trust my body and the feeling of being weak and frail. I became very conscious of the impact sitting was having on my body. The longer I sat the more the pain I felt. It was a simple cause-and-effect relationship that was relieved the moment I stood up and moved even slightly.

Over time I accepted that I was not going to get better without doing the rehab exercises consistently throughout my day and making some fundamental changes in the way I worked and lived. My mindset shifted. I could no longer be sedentary and hope to be truly healthy.

With each visit to the chiropractor, I kept asking myself, "How can I get better? How can I give these rehab exercises a chance?" I also realized that my chiropractor was not aware of how hard it was for me to do the exercises throughout my day at the office. There was no bridge between what she was asking me to do and my ability to do it at work. Our experiences of work were worlds apart.

In her office, she was not sedentary at all: she wore running shoes and was on her feet most of the day moving and adjusting other people's bodies! In her world, movement was natural and logical. In mine movement was strange and unwelcome. It went against the culture of the space; its norms, patterns, and values.

Once I left her office I was on my own with the details of remembering how to do the exercises, how often to do them, and where to do them. I was also on my own to coach myself to stay motivated, to not feel embarrassed, to stay focused, and to hold myself accountable. I realized that moving at the office was a tall order for anyone.

At the time, I thought what was missing for me was support and accountability. The reality was even if my chiropractor was able to follow me around 24/7 giving me guidance and reminders, it still wouldn't have changed the culture of my workplace, nor my attitude about how movement did not belong at the workplace.

I realized that I had to change my relationship with my body regardless of the environment. This could eventually lead to changes between myself, my colleagues, and my environment. I realized that I had to find a way to transform these unspoken rules against movement in the workplace that I had internalized so deeply.

I also realized that the gap I experienced with my chiropractor probably occurred with many people receiving care from physiotherapists, massage therapists, doctors, nutritionists, and other healthcare providers. I saw a need for change for patients, clients, and people that went beyond the doctor's office and into people's daily lives at work and at home. Later I found research that showed the rate of noncompliance to rehab exercises to be as high as 65 percent!

I moved from being a passive recipient of healthcare to an actively engaged pursuer of health. I was not interested in simple recovery. I wanted to be healthy and I wanted to establish a daily practice that would enable me to address sedentary time throughout my entire day. I used my experiences as a personal trainer to organize the exercises into a daily program and my experiences as a therapist to clarify my readiness for change and overcome my resistance to moving at work.

I was ready for change. I absolutely wanted to say goodbye to the pain in my back and take back my health. I decided I would do whatever it took to be healthy at work. I would no longer compromise my health to do a job. I would find a way to work well and be well at the same time.

I set a goal of five rehab exercises a day. I used my iPhone timer to trigger me to do it and my notepad to track what I was doing. Each time I did an exercise, it would take no more than one or two minutes. It was not disruptive to my work at all. In fact, moving was an energizing and refreshing break from staring at the computer screen and being stuck in my head.

Just one month later, the dull ache and soreness in my back was completely gone. During this time, I stopped seeing my chiropractor. I was so impressed by these results I began to incorporate movements such as push ups, planks, squats, and yoga moves throughout my day. My core strength, balance, and flexibility improved dramatically as well as my energy.

With more energy I was more productive at work and my mood improved noticeably. I no longer had an energy drop midafternoon after lunch so I didn't need coffee to wake me up. I told my colleagues, and many of them began to take movement breaks with me.

I kept feeling better the more I moved throughout my day so I brought exercise equipment to work: a resistance band, a kettlebell, a chin-up bar, and a yoga mat. This helped me vary the exercises I could do at work. I even built a standing desk. I no longer felt self-conscious or embarrassed about doing these things at work because I was determined to prioritize my health as the foundation for my work and life. At the same time, I felt energized to do my work. Because I had the confidence of knowing that my health was improving and growing, I was in a positive frame of mind and I felt more capable of handling the stress that inevitably came up at work.

Three months after I injured my back, I had lost 15 pounds. I had always exercised three to four times per week and I made no changes to that or my diet. Now I am at a healthy weight of 172 pounds, which I maintain easily with MOVE breaks spread throughout my day.

I discovered a huge body of research that linked being sedentary to all sorts of health problems: slower metabolism, obesity, cancer, diabetes, poor back health, and lowered mood and focus. The research revealed that even one hour of exercise a day did not offset the negative effects of being sedentary. According to researchers, sitting impacts the body like smoking does regardless if you also eat a salad every day.

As a bodybuilder, I relied on the traditional model of working out an hour a day, but to be healthy I created ThinkMOVE to address the other 15 hours of my waking life. Using the ThinkMOVE method, there is no limit to what goals you can pursue.

Perhaps you are like me and are dealing with a nagging injury and you need time and space to do your rehab exercises, and a system of remembering to do them and track them. The strategies and techniques in this book will help you. Maybe you'd like to be stronger or more flexible, you can easily implement MOVE breaks into your day that will enhance these abilities. In addition to converting sedentary time into opportunities for health, this approach helps people become active participants in their healthcare rather than passive recipients of treatment.

2. Why Is Sitting So Bad?

So what exactly is happening to our bodies when we sit?

- Electrical activity in the leg muscles shut off.

- Calorie burning drops to one calorie per minute (Walking is about three calories per minute).

- Enzymes that help break down fat drop 90 percent, leading to weight gain.

- Good cholesterol drops 20 percent after just two hours of sitting.

- Sitting accelerates the aging process through decreased bone density and muscle atrophy.

The physical effects of sitting occur within a few hours of prolonged sitting. Understanding that the negative physiological effects happen in the short term (just a few hours) can motivate you to find solutions that address these effects. Sitting is having an impact on your metabolism, your heart, your muscles, and your bones right now.

Unfortunately, replacing one stagnant position is not a viable solution. The body adapts. Eventually the solution loses effectiveness. You must learn to incorporate frequent bouts of movement to offset sedentary time. Varying the type of movements will stimulate all the physiological systems of the body that fall asleep while you are sitting.

Through years of training both at school and work, we have imprisoned our bodies into chairs and desks for too long. It's time to free our bodies so they are free to move.

How pervasive are the issues of being sedentary? The average Canadian adults sits nine and a half hours each day. If you're reading this book, your sitting time may exceed this number. In the overall labor force, 80 percent of jobs are almost completely sedentary. When 50 to 70 percent of our daily lives are spent sitting and another 30 percent sleeping, it's easy to understand why getting into gym clothes and doing an intense workout seems so daunting. Statistics show that only 15 percent of adults and seven percent of children are meeting the minimum recommended physical activity guidelines each day. We need to account for our sedentary culture in order to understand why health issues like obesity and chronic illness are so pervasive.

A study by Ian Janssen, Canada Research Chair in physical activity and obesity at Queen's University, found that couch potato lifestyles cost Canadians $6.8 billion in total patient care, workplace absenteeism, and long-term disability.

Research by Dr. Emma Wilmot of the Diabetes Research Group in Britain analyzed 18 studies involving almost 800,000 people. Those who sat the most had a 147 percent increased risk of a heart attack or stroke, 112 percent increase in the risk of developing diabetes, 90 percent greater risk of dying from a cardiac event, and a 49 percent greater risk of premature mortality (all causes). The least active were the most at risk for developing major health complications such as coronary artery disease, stroke, hypertension, colon cancer, breast cancer, Type 2 diabetes, and osteoporosis. Frequent TV and web surfers (sitters) had higher rates of hypertension, obesity, high blood triglycerides and blood sugar, and low HDL cholesterol, regardless of weight.

2.1 It's about movement, not exercise

I make a distinction between movement and exercise. I define traditional exercise as it is defined by researchers, as any acute single daily bout of physical activity that amounts to moderate to vigorous intensity, typically 30 to 60 minutes.

Most marketing efforts that push exercise focus on shaping the body to look a certain way. You don't have to look far to see media depictions of distinct abs, and thin waists beside cars or shampoo products. This approach tends to objectify and alienate us from our bodies. Exercise and sport can have a positive impact on health but often the goals are aesthetic- or performance-based and health is secondary. Most exercise programs promote a kind of hardcore attitude that costs health rather than enhances it, with overtraining and injury. Emphasizing movement over exercise addresses the sedentary issue and creates a clearer, more direct path to health.

Movement in the office and throughout our day is not about achieving a particular aesthetic but moving towards health and enhancing work. If people could begin to focus on incorporating movement into their days and worrying less about exercise time, maybe it would be more acceptable, even normal. You don't need all the mirrors, sweat, or weights to be a healthy human being. You only need to give yourself permission to move.

Does exercise help offset the effects of being sedentary? The short answer is no. Exercise and sedentary time are independent variables just as smoking a cigarette has an impact on your health whether or not you eat salads for lunch every day.

The study by the National Cancer Institute explored whether the impact of prolonged sitting was reduced by exercising. Participants were asked how much time they spent in cars, watching TV, sitting in front of a computer, and exercising. At the beginning of the study none of the participants suffered from heart disease, cancer, or diabetes. After eight years many were ill and died. The most unhealthy tended to be the most sedentary. Exercising an hour daily did not do much to reduce the risk. People who exercised for seven hours or more a week but spent at least five or more hours a day in front of the television were more likely to die prematurely than the group who exercised seven hours a week and watched less than an hour of TV a day.

Even at seven hours of exercise per week — that's 420 minutes more than the 150 minutes recommended by physical activity guidelines —

the startling conclusion was that exercise in any amount even at high frequencies, did not protect against premature death when people were still highly sedentary the rest of the time.

In a related study by the American Cancer Society, the researchers lead by Alpha Patel, PhD, analyzed whether the people who sat watching television had other unhealthy habits that caused them to die sooner. But even after accounting for these other unhealthy habits and analyzing the data, they reported that "age, sex, education, smoking, hypertension, waist circumference, body-mass index, glucose tolerance status and leisure-time exercise did not significantly modify the associations between television viewing (sitting) and all-cause … mortality."

Sitting, he concluded, is an independent pathology. "Being sedentary for nine hours a day at the office is bad for your health whether you go home and watch television afterward or hit the gym. It is bad whether you are morbidly obese or marathon-runner thin ... Several factors could explain the positive association between time spent sitting and higher all-cause death rates," said Dr. Patel. "Prolonged time spent sitting, independent of physical activity, has been shown to have important metabolic consequences, and may influence things like triglycerides, high density lipoprotein, cholesterol, fasting plasma glucose, resting blood pressure, and leptin, which are biomarkers of obesity and cardiovascular and other chronic diseases."

"Excessive sitting is a lethal activity," Dr. James Levine, another leading researcher in this area suggests.

We need to fundamentally rethink the way we live and work. It turns out that exercise alone does not address the problem of being sedentary since sitting is not a benign activity. Paradoxically, inactivity is actively harming your body by increasing risk for heart disease, cancer, diabetes, and obesity.

After trying Exercise 1, reflect on what it might be like to bring this new choice to stand and move at your office as it is now? Do you imagine it would be easy or difficult? What feelings or thoughts or practical considerations would get in the way? It takes time and skill to unlearn what we have spent most of our lives learning to do, which is to sit.

The jury is out on what amount of sitting is okay. Some studies suggest that reducing sitting time to less than three hours per day would increase life expectancy by two years. Another found that for every hour of sitting time a person's life expectancy is reduced by 22 minutes!

While we wait for researchers to figure out how many hours we can tolerate, you can begin to use the ThinkMOVE method to disrupt every hour of sitting time. Frequent disruptions of sedentary time is what matters most; as little as one to three minutes per hour.

Before we can talk about the solution we need to understand some of the barriers that stand in our way. Implementing this program requires transformation of our culture including the way we work, the way we think about movement, and our ideas of health and body image.

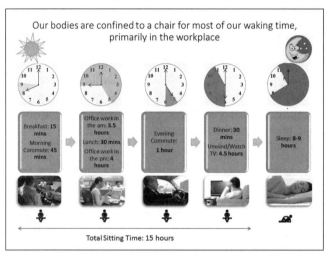

Figure 4

Exercise 1
Take a Stand Against Sitting

Now that you've become aware of some of the adverse effects of sitting, I'd like to invite you try a short experiment.

Imagine you are at work right now. (If you are at work, even better!) Bring yourself to the place where you sit most often. This could be in your office at your desk or if you work in an open concept space, your own workspace. Feel the chair beneath you. See the space and the people in it with all the colors and shapes and sounds. Imagine that you are feeling tired, groggy, sore, and stiff from sitting and you are thinking about all the information you've been learning about and how harmful prolonged sitting can be.

Now imagine simply standing up in the middle of whatever you are doing and taking a break from sitting. Maybe there are people around you. Take a moment to imagine what this would be like. Perhaps if you are sitting now, you can take a moment to stand up and feel what this would be like.

Imagine your muscles activating, your blood flowing against gravity. Take a few deep breaths to help relax and let go of some of the tension you were feeling. Perhaps wiggle or shake your arms, your neck, your hips and your legs to help flush out the stiffness.

Listen carefully to what's happening on the inside. What happens when you imagine taking a moment to listen to your body and doing something good for it while at work? What is happening in your thoughts? In your body? What happens to your senses?

Pay attention to any thoughts or feelings, particularly those of resistance: "This is strange. People will think I'm weird." See if you can listen to what's going on inside your body, your thoughts and feelings. Notice the judgments and let them go for now.

What do you think it would be like to listen to your body within the context of a group? Allow yourself to imagine what might happen for you in relation to yourself, your colleagues, and your environment. Would it help if other people were also standing and moving?

Did you find it difficult to imagine taking a break from sitting when everyone else around was seated? If so, it means you were a good student to what you were taught in school. Sitting still has been the norm and to stand or move is new and different. Naturally this would feel odd.

This exercise is meant to help you become aware of the barriers to movement, both real and imagined. Moving itself is pretty easy. You just stand up and move around. But doing it freely in the context of work can be very difficult. Overcoming our internal resistance to movement is an important ingredient to creating a moving culture. Once many people start to free themselves of imagined restrictions on our bodies we can begin to move freely as a group.

Exercise 2
How Much Do You Sit?

If you reflect on your day, you may recognize there are many opportunities to sit. Take a moment to think about your typical day and calculate the number of hours you sit.

Morning: _____

Commute: _____

Office: _____

Lunch: _____

Office: _____

Commute: _____

Evening: _____   **Total = _____**

2
The Business Case for Movement

On September 2, 2015, Alan Kurdi, a three-year-old Syrian boy, drowned and the image of his body washed ashore made global headlines. The heartbreak of this image woke me up to the Hell on Earth realities facing Syrian refugees. This prompted a conversation with my wife's parents, to hear their refugee story as Vietnamese "boat people" who arrived in Canada in 1980.

My wife had heard bits and pieces of the story growing up, but never one cohesive narrative. We heard about the 35 days her parents spent navigating the rough waters of the South China Sea. How two parents and a four-year-old girl had to survive on only a single cup of water and a bowl of rice each day. How there was only room for women and children to lie down at night in the lower deck while men had to spend the nights sitting and wandering the main deck to protect the boat from pirates. Twenty-one days into the journey there was a breach in the body of the boat and it began to sink. Many who had taken this risky journey died, but fortunately for my wife's parents, a Chinese fishing boat noticed their cries for help and towed them safely to shore. They arrived in Hong Kong a few weeks later where they lived for a year as refugees before coming to Canada.

What stood out to me in hearing their story and observing their lives was the power of community that enabled them to survive such overwhelming odds. I had a deeper understanding within the context of their refugee story of why they were so loyal to their friends and why they pushed us so hard to invite 200 of their friends to our wedding when we only wanted 100 people total.

Their sacrifice and courage was humbling to me in ways I couldn't express adequately. As they spoke, a wave of intense gratitude and awe washed over me as if I was meeting these people for the very first time.

After 30 years, they are still connected to their friends who left Vietnam. They share food from their gardens, attend each other's children's weddings, and celebrate successes. They lived the idea of "rising tides lift all boats" and have been a powerful example for my wife and myself of the importance of family and community.

In our modern society, specifically in urban centers in North America, we chase things like job titles and bonuses. We want the latest gadgets and always a little bit more money. But are these things the most important pursuits? I wonder what is at the heart of our efforts.

The emphasis on movement in this book is really a movement towards actualizing our true health potential within and through our communities. The Vietnamese refugees fled their homeland in search of freedom and a joyful life. When my wife's parents arrived in Canada, they were happy to have work and accepted back-breaking labor to pay the rent and put food on the table for their children. Within their communities, they helped each other find jobs, raised each other's children, and renovated each other's homes.

Businesses have opportunity to create communities of people happy to show up at work and be enthusiastically engaged in the mission and vision of the companies. We can learn lessons from the Vietnamese boat people about the importance of building communities if we recognize that the places we go to work every day are our communities.

We can increase the quality of our lives if we take a communal approach to health and well-being in addition to our conventionally individualistic approach, where we only talk about health matters privately with our doctors, health professionals, or personal trainers. Of course, many health issues are private. However, issues like sedentarism, food choices, and workload are all relevant to the workplace.

The actualization of health and living well is our collective inheritance and responsibility, which has been built on the hard work and sacrifice of the previous generation. We can continue this evolution if we focus on improving the quality of our workplaces, where we spend a majority of our waking hours, which includes things like cost savings and increasing productivity, but more importantly our experience of health, connection, growth, and fulfillment.

Incorporating health at the workplace means that people as a community are making the choice every day to care for themselves and each other. Genuine care goes well beyond abstract notions of numbers and money. Caring means asking, "How are you?" and listening. As long as workplaces focus on the number as a way of attracting and retaining talent, employees will be loyal to the extent that they are paid.

The true basis for loyalty is not money, but relationships. When I look around at people in my generation, the Millennials, it is quite common for people to change jobs every year or two. People are looking for jobs that are challenging and fulfilling and provide support to do a great job, and that provide opportunities to be healthy. Unless organizations find ways to care about employees' physical and mental health, people will continue their secret job searches.

This chapter is written for the human resources professional, business owner, executive, or manager interested in understanding the business case for movement. ThinkMOVE is an opportunity to create a community through the pursuit of health. By practicing physical movement, people learn to take care of themselves and to support one another. This chapter can also help the employee who would like to be a champion at work for health programs like ThinkMOVE that encourage movement at their workplace.

1. To Be Profitable and Sustainable, You Need Health

Money or health: Which is more important? I often think about the life of Steve Jobs. It's clear that by the end of his life, more time would be worth more than any amount of money. As the saying goes, time is money. If we have health, it's more likely we have time.

In 2008, the financial markets crashed. After a long period of steady financial growth, companies were hitting their numbers, but not as concerned with sustainability. The short-sighted greed for more money lead to a collective neglect of doing what was sustainable and the result was the worst recession since the Great Depression.

We've seen what hyper-focusing on profit can look like, but knowing how to be sustainable and profitable is a more complex problem. It demands that the needs of all people impacted by a company be considered: owners, employees, and customers. Helping employees work in ways that are healthy is an important part of building a sustainable business that can also build long term profits. Because, when it comes to health, there is always a cost to neglecting it.

As it turns out, working a sedentary office job can be hazardous to one's health. As we have explored, the cumulative damage of prolonged sitting to one's metabolism, immune system, musculoskeletal health, and heart health results in lowered quality of life and healthcare costs in the billions. Prioritizing health isn't just about lowering costs related to sickness and burnout. Before money, we need the resource of health that makes work and profit possible.

All this seems obvious, but common sense does not mean common practice. I've encountered too many companies caught up in old patterns of working at the expense of health instead of working with health. A good place to start is by asking: Are we working in ways that make us healthier or unhealthier?

Many companies have unconsciously adopted unhealthy ways of working inherited from previous generations. A workaholic attitude combined with anti-health practices like working long hours, eating junk food, skipping sleep, skipping meals, and taking cigarette breaks have been the model of successful careers.

Working in ways that are sustainable for health is a path to sustainable profit growth. Simon Sinek, in his book *Leaders Eat Last*, cites the example of Costco as a company that focuses on long-term, sustainable growth by taking care of its people. This approach has resulted in Costco's stocks making steady and predictable progress over the long term.

People are less willing to work towards a retirement. As Tim Ferriss calls it: the Deferred-Life Plan. Millennials and many others are in search of work that gives them a fulfilling experience of life today. Health needs to be a part of that picture and is a critical dimension of meaningful and fulfilling work experiences.

Working in ways that are sustainable to health means finding creative and innovative ways of working that honor the moment-to-moment health needs of the body.

A healthy workplace is one where people are able to manage their energy so they feel autonomous, relationships between people feel respectful, and people are able to take care of their bodies by having the freedom to move and make healthy choices for themselves.

Health matters can be pushed into the shadows for only so long. Eventually our bodies come out of the darkness in the form of a nightmare such as long-term illness or disability.

You can begin the conversation with your team with the question: Are we working in ways that make us healthier or unhealthier? The next step would be clearly defining ways that the entire company can practice healthier ways of working that are sustainable. I would recommend starting small and slowly with these changes. Changing the way people work requires surgical precision since people have been conditioned to work in habitual ways, particularly in a sedentary manner and often have reasonable concerns about being judged or left out when it comes to their health. Health initiatives should always be voluntary; invitations rather than rigid expectations.

Exercise 3 offers three micro-health changes that leaders in organizations can use to begin the journey of creating a healthy and sustainable workforce. Others can share these as suggestions with their boss.

Exercise 3
Move during the Day

1. **MOVE breaks:** Incorporate two movement-based breaks a day. One mid-morning (10:00 a.m.) and one midafternoon (3:00 p.m.). Invite colleagues to take five minutes to connect and do some light stretches. Get re-energized and back to work.

2. **A 30-second health check-in:** Take 30 seconds every day to ask: What's one small thing I can do for my health? Think low time/energy output. Examples are: drink more water, take the stairs, five deep breaths.

3. **Learn to say "no" and ask for help:** Type-A people will resist this, but one of the unhealthiest patterns at work is the compulsion to say yes to everything and not recognize and respect one's limitations. Being able to say "no" or "I need help" is a part of being productive and healthy.

These suggestions are simple and take very little time, but they are not easy. They require commitment and action. Pick one item that seems most realistic for you and share with at least one other person your intention to practice this healthy behavior. You might invite him or her to try one too and you can support and encourage each other along the way.

---

2. Leaders Need to Lead with Care First and Cost Second

In order for a health and wellness program to be successful, business owners and leaders need to genuinely care about the health and well-being of their people. They need to be able to see the faces and bodies that are connected to their work community before they see the numbers. When companies approach health and wellness superficially, employees do not take these initiatives seriously and do not engage. As a result, investments in wellness initiatives become a waste of time and money.

In my experience, companies that purchased a wellness program for employees, but whose executive teams did not participate, did not achieve consistent engagement across the organization. Feedback from participants included, "Because I didn't see my director doing it, I didn't feel like it was a priority or that I should be taking the time to do it for myself."

Many companies invest primarily in benefit packages for their employees that focus on treatment (e.g., chiropractor, physiotherapy, massage, drugs, etc.). These benefits are meant to attract and retain talented employees and to provide a sense of security. Logically, a treatment-only strategy leaves employees vulnerable to getting sick in the first place because there is no strategy to build up their health.

Benefits are things that employees typically feel that they need to take advantage of before they run out. I have witnessed many times people making use of their massage therapy benefits before the end of the fiscal year just because they have them.

It would make sense for companies to balance their investments in treatment-based approaches with health and wellness programs that prevent illness and injury from happening in the first place. These wellness programs can reduce cost and enhance employee well-being so they have more energy, feel stronger, and are more connected at work.

A wellness program reduces the risk for illness and injury while enhancing employee engagement, energy, and productivity. When employers and employees participate together, a community of care is built around the health of each person in the company. What people are being invited to do through each move break is to return to their bodies and practice the freedom to move in their work environment. This requires a sense of safety at all levels of the organization.

When a group is able to move together freely, you can be sure that they have achieved a level of safety with each other that they are able to care for their health with energy and confidence, which elevates the tide of health for everyone.

Each employee has the responsibility to genuinely engage wellness initiatives with commitment and a seriousness that acknowledges how important their well-being is, not only to themselves but to the community of work as a whole. Each employee helps contribute to the overall culture of wellness at the workplace. This means, for example, participating as much as they are able and avoiding judgments or teasing of coworkers for the choices they make, healthy or otherwise. Respect and acceptance of others for their choices and readiness for healthy behaviors is an important factor for companies trying to incorporate a wellness initiative.

Establishing the Freedom to Move principle at the workplace represents a transformative shift towards health; one that shows a deep respect and care for each person in the organization. The principle can be manifested in one simple statement from the leaders of a company:

> You have permission to move and take care of your bodies at work by whatever means necessary as long as you do not infringe on other people's rights and your responsibilities to the company.

When it comes to being sedentary, it's not enough for employers to make this statement and then sit ten or more hours a day. CEOs and the management team can be important leaders who model the permission they give others by giving it to themselves. By caring for their own health and modeling healthy movement to the best of their abilities, leaders embody healthy ways of working and join the challenge of actualizing health rather than denying or ignoring it.

By participating in the ThinkMOVE program, employers and employees alike increase energy and internal resources which increases their capacity to be of service to clients and customers.

> Imagine a situation where Maria, a market research analyst, needs to call a client to let them know an error was made on a report and she needs another day to make the corrections. She takes a moment to notice the tension that has been building up in her body all morning and decides to do a stretch and some deep breathing to move through the tension. After taking a minute, she shakes off the nervous energy and explains the situation to the client in a clear and honest way rather than communicating out of fear. Her ability to be calm helped the client remain calm and accept the situation. He was appreciative that she was honest and able to catch the mistake. Maria was able to do the best she could with the situation she faced.

A healthy workforce will inevitably reduce costs associated with illness, disease, and injury. In addition, a comprehensive wellness initiative increases talent retention, recruitment, and engagement. People are more aware of the impact of work on their health. The expectation is that work should be fulfilling and not a source of disease.

3. Practicing Movement at Work Is About Making Choices and Reacting Less

As in the example of Maria, the practice of movement and listening to the body's sensations throughout the day empowers people to use the information absorbed by their bodies. Being professional typically means keeping emotions out of the workplace. It is important to maintain composure and speak in a respectful manner at all times, but denial of emotions is unhealthy. The ThinkMOVE program outlined in this book will teach you a way of staying in touch with yourself so that you can be aware of what it is you are feeling and needing and how to make choices to address those needs.

Energy and emotions need a way to be expressed. Sometimes that might be through some kind of movement or through breath. At other times, movement and breath might help people understand what they need so they can communicate calmly and intelligently. This encourages self-awareness and reduces the reactivity that looks like unhealthy coping, such as shutting down when problems arise.

We need to discard old notions of professionalism that are non-human. Just because people are in the workplace does not mean they don't feel things or have social-emotional needs. We all come with our own psychology, including fears and insecurities, and acknowledging our humanness is an important step towards actualizing health.

A company's vision needs to include employees' well being. If their health is neglected, employees end up burning out and suffering from chronic illnesses, absenteeism, or working at limited capacity. Employees will sacrifice their health, as many of us have learned to do, for the sake of getting work done and meeting their numbers. Unfortunately, this is not an inspiring vision for work, but rather the stress-filled mechanical workplaces a majority of people face daily.

We can all begin to contribute to the health shift in business culture. This begins by playing the long game: Doing the right thing, which means caring about your employees, your colleagues, and yourself. Practice encouraging one another to move, to eat lunch, to connect, to learn new skills, to communicate, to help, and to laugh. By investing time, money, and energy in employee health, a natural reciprocal dynamic occurs. People begin to feel part of a community, not just a company, and will work to contribute to that community.

Movement is a method for engaging employees and creating a culture that will transform a business from numbers-focused to people-focused; from diseased to healthy; from disconnection to connection; from surviving to thriving; from short-term profit to long-term sustainability.

Wellness and work performance are linked. Moving throughout the day isn't just about improving health, but also creating a culture that values wellness and elevates it as the foundation for excellent performance. Engagement and health are closely linked. You can imagine a feedback loop between them, indicating a circular relationship.

4. The Four Business Drivers for Incorporating Healthy Movement in the Workplace

There are four distinct business drivers for creating healthy workplaces:

1. **Financial costs:** These relate to absenteeism and presenteeism and result in healthcare costs as well as productivity losses.

2. **Organizational profile:** The company's reputation, which is relevant to its ability to attract and retain talented employees and the way it fulfills social responsibilities to the larger community. Instead of organizational profile, I will focus on the concept of organizational health, which views the organization as an organic system that can function in a healthy way in the same manner that a human body can function as a healthy system.

3. **Legal case:** An IAPA report (The Business Case for a Healthy Workplace IAPA [Industrial Accident Prevention Association], 2008) summarizes several legal cases where the disregard of employee health resulted in large settlements due to the mental/physical suffering of employees. Corporations have a responsibility to take steps to prevent any harm to employee health.

4. **Productivity:** Unlike other Corporate Wellness approaches, MOVE breaks aren't a break from work that improves work. ThinkMOVE is a way of working that is enhanced. Integrating movement into the flow of one's day can increase energy, focus, and connection.

Let's explore examples to illustrate these business drivers, which are compositions of real life cases.

Case A: Hayden

Hayden, a 43-year-old sales manager is 30 pounds overweight and has been working at Company X for ten years. His day is mostly spent sedentary in meetings, driving, going out for client lunches, answering phone calls, and completing his paperwork. One day he reaches for a file on an upper shelf and pulls his back badly. This injury is a result of his spine being put in a compromised sitting position for more than ten hours a day and his entire body being injury-prone from lack of movement. He makes one sudden movement and suffers a severe low back strain. He misses one day of work, which according to his salary of $100,000 is valued at $381. He misses two sales meetings and needs to reschedule. Hopefully this doesn't compromise the sales.

For the next two weeks he needs to take a third of his work days to visit a chiropractor twice a week for treatments. Each treatment costs $65, and given his $500 company benefits package limit it only takes him three and half weeks to run out of money. Over the course of just one month the company has missed, in total, four working days from Hayden, which means the company continues to pay his salary, approximately $1,500, while getting no work output because Hayden is having to receive treatment.

The benefits package also covers physiotherapy and massage therapy and Hayden, not wanting to pay for treatment out of his own pocket, tries to utilize all the treatment modalities at his disposal. He follows a similar course of treatment frequency as with his chiropractic care for the next two months until both treatment options run out at their limits of $500 each. He continues to miss a third to half a day for his appointments, which costs the company $1,500 towards his salary again, without calculating losses associated with reduced client interaction and sales relevant to Hayden's position.

Typically, each healthcare professional would be recommending rehab exercises that Hayden should be doing throughout his day (once every one to two hours) to disrupt sedentary time and to rehabilitate his back, but Hayden does not comply with this part of his treatment since, like 70 percent of patients, he does not comply with the rehab exercise component of treatment.

His back pain has subsided slightly but it has not stopped. Hayden has begun to take Oxycontin, which costs $4 a pill. He takes three a day to cope with the pain. The cost is covered by the company's drug plan and costs $1,080 in only three months.

The total costs in this example, including Hayden's salary costs due to missed work, treatment, and medication costs, amounts to $7,080 over the course of only three to six months. Losses in this case are significant. The costs to the business as a result of Hayden's absence from the office have not been calculated, but it's clear that client relations would be compromised due to missed meetings and communication. Some sales that would have typically been closed are lost or delayed, pushing those accounts into the next quarter. Other employees would need to support Hayden in his absence and that would put extra pressure on their workload, and contribute negatively to work/life balance.

5. The Financial Cost of Sitting

As Hayden's case illustrates, financial costs associated with physical injury can skyrocket depending on the individual's health history and the outcomes of treatment. When these expenses occur across a proportion of employees, the expenses can cripple a business.

Absenteeism costs are productivity losses that occur when employees are not well enough to work, as well as overtime and overstaffing expenses needed to cover these absences. In the US, studies show that wellness programs reduce healthcare costs by an average of $3.27 for every dollar invested and absenteeism costs drop by $2.73 for every dollar spent. They also estimated that absenteeism-related expenses are as high as $74 billion annually in the US (Lowe, 2014) and in Canada, $3.5 billion annually (IAPA, 2008).

Another factor that increases costs related to health is presenteeism. The case of Hayden is an example. He was not well but showed up to work in a compromised state. In the US alone, costs due to presenteeism are estimated at $150 billion annually (Lowe, 2014).

An unhealthy workplace can result in a variety of costly events such as staff turnover, litigation, decreased employee engagement, absenteeism, health insurance claims, presenteeism, short- and long-term disability, depression and other mental illnesses, and accidents. Each of the items has significant costs, and contributes to decreased productivity.

Addressing the sedentary issue through the ThinkMOVE program is an approach that can reduce the risk and costs associated with illness and injury. The approach can also significantly increase employee engagement by providing a fun and energizing way of working that accounts for the needs of the body while increasing work productivity. Participants in the ThinkMOVE program say that the top benefits they experience are increases in energy, and reductions in body tension, soreness, and pain.

6. The Benefits of Movement on Organizational Health

Using the principles and techniques of ThinkMOVE (more in Chapter 6), a healthy workplace is sustainable. The organization empowers its people to grow and thrive over the long term. By employers modeling genuine care, employees are supported to embody genuine care with clients and customers.

A company that gives employees the Freedom to Move implicitly trusts those people to be responsible and reasonable with their choices. Those employees are empowered to do their best rather than needing to be managed with fear or punishments.

The practice of the ThinkMOVE program empowers the company to not just talk the talk of health, but to put their values into action by creating space for health during the workday. Rather than health practices being restricted to the space of health clinics and gyms, employers provide employees with the skills, resources, and space to practice the Freedom to Move at work.

By addressing prolonged sitting, organizations can transform their work culture to one that is authentically healthy through concrete actions. The organization learns how to work in ways that take into account the needs of the bodies.

Movement Enhancing Work

Mary Ann, the CEO of a mental health company, explained that she and her team were stuck on a specific problem that they could not get their heads around. Tried as they may to think through the issue the team kept getting stuck. Finally, they decided to take a cardio MOVE break and did a minute of desk jogging. They were buzzing and laughing as they got up and moved. Shortly after the break they found a solution to the problem. She explained, "I realized that what we needed wasn't more thinking, but a way of coming back to our bodies and allowing our team to move through the issue."

Moving doesn't just lower the healthcare costs associated with a sedentary lifestyle. There is net psychosocial gain from having the Freedom to Move throughout the day. Imagine buying an insurance policy that covers your costs, but then also pays you out with bonuses along the way enriching your life with health, energy, vitality, and connection.

- Movement doesn't just save the company money, it makes money by improving employee performance at work.

- Movement doesn't just prevent illness, it makes employees healthier, stronger, smarter, friendlier, and happier.

- Movement helps create connections and an overall community that values health and well-being.

- Movement of the body also creates movement of the mind, openness, creativity, and innovation in employees.

Transforming your work culture from sedentary to one that holds space for healthy movement enables people to experience well-being at and through work. Health becomes part of the work day rather than a practice that needs to exist outside the work environment.

Having a comprehensive health and wellness program is not just another perk. It is essential. It enhances work by providing the effects of more energy, reduced pain, and an enhanced way of working.

Case B: Brenda

Brenda is a 28-year-old product manager who suffered from periods of depression in college. She is sensitive to the stress of others and works at a very high-paced, high-stress tech startup. She reports to a director with a punitive and bullying style. Her director continually puts down her work and suggests that she doesn't have enough ambition and is what some would call a "typical Millennial" who isn't willing to put in the work. Her boss' style of management encourages competition and results in distrust between employees. Morale and trust at the office is therefore low and there is no one in whom Brenda trusts enough to confide.

Brenda has been there for almost a year and she feels her nerves have been shot given the pressure and the shaming tactics. She's been asked to work later and later and this has been an ongoing trend. She has no time for exercise and eats poorly whenever she does have the chance to eat.

Her boyfriend has become concerned about her as she has been expressing severe depressive thoughts related to not wanting to wake up in the morning, since there isn't anything to look forward to. He is also concerned about the treatment Brenda is receiving from her director and feels that it borders on abusive behavior. Overall, Brenda is suffering from low feelings of self-worth and is barely able to make it through a workday. She is tempted to drink in the evenings as a way to relieve some of the stress, but given a history of alcoholism in his family her boyfriend has tried his best to avoid this.

Since her performance has been degrading significantly over the past month, she is concerned that she will be fired as others at the company have been let go for underperforming.

Her boyfriend is encouraging her to speak to a lawyer to possibly file a wrongful dismissal suit if this happens. Brenda has been seeing a psychotherapist for the past month and she meets criteria for major depressive disorder. Brenda is open to speaking with a lawyer and wants to be prepared in case she is fired.

She would like to find another job but given her current health condition she does not possess the motivation or energy to pursue a job search. Overall, she feels quite hopeless about her situation and feels highly resentful towards the company and her director.

This case illustrates the negative impacts a toxic work culture can have on mental health. Unbeknownst to the company, it is highly vulnerable to legal action due to the unreasonable workload and harassment resulting in Brenda's mental distress. A high-profile lawsuit would have obvious negative implications for the company's public profile as well as negative impacts on the morale of the current staff. The costs in cases like Brenda's can range in the millions of dollars. The blatant disregard for reasonable human limitations and dignity have progressively worse impacts on not only Brenda's productivity but the company as a whole. When a work environment is this toxic, the effect on health and productivity is exponential rather than gradual.

7. The Benefits of a Healthy Work Culture

Until we can address health within our communities, not just as individuals, and in particular the workplace where we spend most of our time, we will be stuck in treatment models of healthcare, not fulfilling our potential. Living and working in a healthy way is an important consideration for both employers and employees. Healthy ways of working serve the organization, clients/customers, and the community at large. It is the socially responsible thing to do because raising a generation of unhealthy employees creates a tremendous burden on future generations not only in terms of healthcare costs and the demand for familial caregiving, but also by perpetuating unhealthy ways of working to the next generation.

Health requires communal efforts. The patterns of the group at work and at home become our ingrained behavioral patterns. Whether we move or sit all day, or eat healthy or unhealthy foods is largely determined by the patterns of the majority.

8. Productivity: Movement Isn't a Break from Working, It Is a Way of Working

Some companies are at a stage where they want to enhance their profile by having perks like a gym, or healthy lunches, but this misses the mark of what is powerful about movement. It's not just a cost-saving strategy or a profile-enhancer. Movement is a method of working and working well. One that enhances the quality of work and the quality of the work experience, which over time become one and the same.

The approach presented in this book is not just about moving for the purpose of addressing the negative physical effects of being sedentary (though it certainly does that). What we do with our bodies, the way we embody our consciousness, impacts every level of our experience whether it's psychological, social, or organizational.

You can do MOVE exercises lasting just a minute to transition into work, as a break to restore your energy, as a way to connect with colleagues, or as a way of transitioning out of work and into home life. Our bodies are the means through which we experience life, so it makes sense to account for the needs of our bodies and to learn to use our bodies optimally throughout every moment of the day.

Moving the body generates tremendous energy and power. What you will learn in the rest of this book is a method of incorporating short breaks of movement lasting between 30 seconds to two minutes that increases body awareness, flexibility, balance, strength, and cardio. Each of these has the power to help improve the quality of work by calming the mind, reducing tension and stress, or increasing energy and focus.

Part of this challenge of ThinkMOVE is that as individuals practice listening to and becoming more aware of their bodies' needs throughout the day, they will have a deeper understanding when things are not going well. This could mean specific organizational issues related to disengagement and job dissatisfaction. Being aware of these issues is a positive first step. It then becomes the choice of the employee to express his or her needs to the appropriate person. It is up to leaders of the organization to create a safe space for this dialogue to happen.

Transforming the environmental context including our social surroundings is vital for behavioral change. Imagine trying to quit smoking when all your coworkers, friends, and family smoke. Smoking is one of the most difficult habits to break, but with all the new bylaws and the overall social stigma associated with smoking, quitting and staying away from cigarettes is much easier today than it was 30 years ago. Now if "sitting is the new smoking" we may be at the beginning steps of creating the conditions to make sitting for ten hours a day as unacceptable as smoking is today. Leveraging the power that our social context can have on us can make it easier to overcome individual impulsivity, self-control challenges, habitual learning, and emotional patterns.

What will help companies survive and thrive in the future is their ability to remain innovative and to grow in the face of rapidly changing times. I argue that it's not primarily more or better technology that is going to provide the business edge, but an evolved way of staying connected to our bodies at work. One that takes us from the trapped and disembodied positions of sitting, to fluid and creative movement that helps us get connected with ourselves and each other so we can feel healthy and joyful, in turn enhancing productivity and the bottom line.

What's fulfilling for people is a question best left to those responsible for setting the missions and visions for their specific companies. What I will say is that incorporating the Freedom to Move in your workplace will help empower people to actualize that vision because people will have access to their health and energy in ways that are not possible if they are disconnected from their bodies. It is important work to help generations of workers understand how an organization's mission is directly related to each individual's well-being.

3

Transforming the Sedentary Work Culture

- "I'm so busy with work I haven't even had a chance to eat lunch!"
- "I'm so busy I haven't even gone to the bathroom!"
- "I'm so busy I haven't worked out in months!"
- "I'm so busy I don't have time to cook."
- "I'm so busy I don't even sleep!"
- "My back is sore from sitting and working nonstop!"

Does any of this sound familiar?

I have experienced work cultures where neglecting one's health is the norm. I have noticed the unspoken pride my colleagues and I seemed to have around our suffering, as if neglecting health were a badge of honor. There was an odd camaraderie, and maybe a subtle competition, built around how unhealthy we were becoming for the sake of our work. It seemed like skipping lunch, water, or exercise somehow made you more productive, dedicated, or committed. I noticed that people in leadership tended to model this way of being productive, that is, work with blatant disregard for their health.

I had internalized this attitude to the detriment of my health. As a result, I noticed weight gain, frequent sickness, lowered mood, and fatigue. It was clearly not a sustainable way of working or living and certainly not something deserving of pride.

Why is being unhealthy so strongly reinforced? If we are searching for ways to be truly healthy then it makes sense to seriously reconsider the state of our health in the place we spend most of our time. Making sustainable changes at work throughout our day can have the greatest impact on our physical and mental well-being, when compared to a few hours spent at the gym or a few months spent on the newest fad diet.

A negligent stance towards health will continue to make health and work incompatible. Instead of being at odds with one another, we need to understand that health is the incredible resource that makes work possible and when health stops, work stops. In order to make that shift, we must transform our beliefs and core values and see the workplace as an important factor in our level of health.

Whether it's sitting too much, not exercising enough, or eating unhealthy foods, many of our explanations about why people fail to be healthy often focus on blaming the individual. As a personal trainer, I heard over and over again people blaming themselves: I don't have enough time, willpower, or money. It was always about the individual not having or being enough. My clients carried around a lot of guilt and shame regarding the state of their health. Most often they would talk about their commitment to work as taking up a majority of their time and energy until finally they had reached the point where they were diagnosed with serious heart conditions or diabetes.

By moving away from blaming the individual, we can empower ourselves to make new choices and work together to transform the context so it is more supportive of our health. Cultural influences on an individual's behavior include specific work cultures, as well as our sedentary habits, traditional models of exercise, media depictions of ideal body types, and advances in technology. These factors interact in ways that can make living a healthy lifestyle extremely challenging.

In the next section, we'll take a closer look at each factor, moving away from thinking about health strictly as a ME problem but also a WE challenge. By attending to the group dynamics, you will increase the likelihood of implementing the exercises and techniques in this book. In order to be sustainable, we need to partner with our environment and others to create health transformations.

1. Our Sedentary Ways and the Traditional Model of Exercise

Our culture sends us conflicting messages about how we should work and take care of our bodies. At school, we are taught to sit still and not fidget. This continues when we start working and we become even more sedentary at the office. Making it up the corporate ladder means getting to that corner office with a larger desk and an even comfier chair!

At the same time, we are bombarded with images telling us we should look like athletes, models, or actors who have no connection to our daily sedentary reality. On the one hand, we are encouraged to train so we can attain the media's ideal of a beautiful, healthy body, even while our workaholic culture and busy lifestyles have us sitting all day neglecting our health. This double message makes it difficult, if not impossible, to know what to do.

The problem is in the overall picture, not the individual parts. We don't need another exercise program to replace INSANITY®. We need to find ways to integrate how we work and take care of our health rather than living in a way that separates the two. The way we currently do both contributes to many of the health problems we see today: obesity, heart disease, diabetes, back pain, osteoporosis to name a few.

In the next chapter, we will show the science of how ThinkMOVE combines working well with being well in an evidence-based, supportive, sustainable, and time sensitive way. You will be invited to rethink traditional forms of exercise and prioritize your time and energy towards movement. The approach that is being suggested here is movement that stems from self-awareness of one's whole body, rather than external prescriptions of exercises and how you should look.

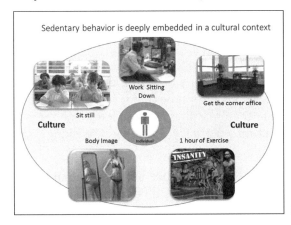

Figure 5

2. Current Solutions Actually Create Barriers to Health

When we were more involved in the physical as part of our daily work, whether it was hunting, farming, or factory work, our bodies received plenty of meaningful physical activity. The idea of exercising in a gym or in your living room to a DVD would have seemed absurd to someone who just finished toiling in the fields for 14 hours!

In the last hundred years, we have successfully engineered physical activity out of our daily lives. Because of this, exercise has become the primary way of adding movement to our lives, but it doesn't change the fact that we are still very sedentary.

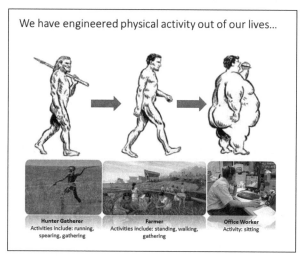

We have engineered physical activity out of our lives...

Hunter Gatherer
Activities include: running, spearing, gathering

Farmer
Activities include: standing, walking, gathering

Office Worker
Activity: sitting

Figure 6

3. Rethinking Exercise: Who Has Time to Exercise, Anyway?

Exercise can feel like having a part-time job. You travel to the gym, change your outfit, do your workout, then shower, change, and travel home. This takes up a lot of time that is separated from the rest of our lives; whereas in the past, physical exertion was integrated seamlessly in our work and into our daily chores (e.g., walking, washing clothes, chopping wood).

It's unrealistic to expect office workers who aren't in the habit of paying attention to their bodies all day to turn on a switch and work out after sitting for ten hours straight. Don't get me wrong, I love to exercise. I have been training since I was 15, but one thing I realized once I started working in an office is our model of fitness isn't for everyone and I repeat: Exercise does not offset the effects of sedentary time.

Research shows that only 15 percent of the population is meeting the minimum recommended 150 minutes a week of moderate to vigorous physical activity — exercising in the traditional sense. A considerable amount of the evidence in support of the 150-minutes-per-week recommendation suggests further that the 150 minutes should be spread across at least five days per week.

That means that a whopping 95 percent of the population has not found consistent success with the conventional model of exercise. This begs the question: If 95 percent of people are failing to meet daily recommended activity guidelines, isn't it the case that the solutions we have are inadequate? To make matters worse, since traditional exercise does nothing to make us less sedentary throughout the day, we can conclude that they are inadequate. The high rate of failure with traditional forms of exercise (95 percent failure rate) has implications for the general population as a whole.

Given these statistics, I'm sure many of you can relate to the common experience of starting and stopping an exercise program, purchasing a gym membership that you never use, buying exercise DVDs that you don't watch, or storing exercise equipment that is now collecting dust. These repeated failures chip away at our confidence that we can be in charge of our bodies and become healthy. We can have compassion for the sedentary corporate employee frozen in the seated position who is challenged to engage in an exercise program. Understanding the context, it makes sense why it is so difficult to motivate a person to exercise.

After so many failed attempts, people get to a point where they feel like giving up on their health because they feel they're not meeting society's expectations for exercise. This often results in individuals making conclusions about their identities which further disconnects them from their bodies:

- "I'm too lazy to work out."
- "It's too late. Who cares how much more weight I put on now?"
- "I have no willpower."
- "I'm hopeless."

- "I just don't have the time."
- "I hate exercise and exercise hates me."

Accompanying these negative self-beliefs are feelings of guilt, shame, helplessness, and disappointment about their relationship to their bodies and their overall health. Because these feelings are internalized in the individual it's difficult to take a step back and see the influence of culture and the larger factors that contribute to the situation.

The repeated experiences of failure, guilt, shame, and helplessness create a wall of resistance to thinking about health. For many people, once that wall of resistance is built, it is not until they get diagnosed with diabetes, a heart condition or experience significant weight gain that they try again. The barrier to entry for non-exercisers and sedentary office workers who have put on a few pounds is not helped by the intimidation factor of many gyms and fitness programs.

With people being so busy with their careers and raising a family, many people wonder:

- "How can I exercise when I have no time?"
- "Will I even be able to do the exercises/workouts? I'm so out of shape! I don't want to be embarrassed!"
- "Will I be able to sustain my efforts and keep up with the program in the long term?"

You can throw out those feelings of helplessness, disappointment, guilt, and shame about exercise by making movement your primary aim. Movement is accessible for everyone.

Begin right now. If it's possible, stand up and walk to the nearest window (aim for 30 seconds to your destination) and come back. That's a one-minute MOVE break! Even if you are stuck in your seat you can wiggle your fingers, shake your legs and turn your neck. You can breathe deeply expanding your lungs and creating space between your ribs, sitting up taller with each breath. When it comes to exercise, it's easy to get stuck in what you can't do. With movement, there are endless possibilities of what you *can* do.

The ThinkMOVE program helps address many of the barriers to exercise by weaving health practices into the layers of corporate culture, physical environment, relationships, and mindset. We remove time as a barrier to health by helping organizations normalize movement at work in short bouts, and to see movement as a work enhancer.

The focus is less on doing the right things and more on letting the simplicity of body awareness combined with movement be the path to being healthy. ThinkMOVE transforms the expectation that to get into shape you need to go to the gym. The reality is, you don't.

Let me repeat that: You absolutely do not have to go to a gym to be fit and healthy. With short breaks and simple movements that anyone can do incorporated into your day, you can disrupt sedentary time and increase your cumulative physical activity time. You can work well and improve your health anywhere and anytime. By meeting people where they are, successful change and goal attainment is far more likely than a fitness program that is disconnected from a person's daily reality. The ThinkMOVE approach is a new model of health and wellness that addresses both the sedentary time and the need for exercise by focusing on movement in all its varieties. It is designed for the 95 percent of people who struggle to add exercise to their day and for anyone who spends most of the day sitting, whether they exercise regularly or not.

4. The Culture of Ideal Body Images

The rise of body image consciousness and weight obsession has grown with the flood of media depictions of athletic, muscular, and toned bodies with very low body fat. Ideal body types are constantly changing. Along with them the various fad products, workouts, and diets promising to help people achieve that ideal. Almost every exercise program uses the ubiquitous "before and after" technique to demonstrate how effective they are at making people look healthier. This assumes that weight is the primary measure of health, but that is only part of the story.

Everyone experiences health differently. Have you considered your own picture of a healthy you? Beyond how you might look, consider how would you feel if you were truly healthy. How would you feel during the normal events of daily living that include children, groceries, stairs? What beliefs and attitudes would you have towards yourself and your body? How would your various body parts feel from the inside out? Consider all your incredible senses, limbs, joints, and muscles. It is empowering to begin to define health outside of cultural norms.

Unfortunately, our models for health are literally models in magazines, actors in movies, or professional athletes. These celebrities often market their products directly to us. So, we try to do what they do to look how they look. Now I'm not arguing against looking good and feeling great about your physical appearance, but when an entire industry is obsessed with image it becomes easy to lose sight of health. I experienced this when I transitioned from being a personal trainer to a full-time, chair-bound therapist. I had no idea that sitting was slowly putting me at risk for a back injury. At the time I had no idea how to address these problems within the workplace.

Achieving an ideal body image may symbolize health and vitality in our current culture, but what does health look like beyond the layers of skin and beyond gym walls? How does a healthy person feel within his or her body during a day at the office or in the home?

In Chapter 7, Health Defined, I'll share a definition that sees health as a resource that enables us to do the things we love with the people we love. This may help you move beyond image-based ideals of health and increase your appreciation for all the things that your current state of health enables you to do, and learn how increasing your health resource will empower you that much further.

5. Advances in Technology and the Mind/Body Chasm

When we were hunters or farmers, our minds and bodies were integrated as one fluid whole and engaged as such throughout the day (see Figure 7). Higher cognitive processes (strategizing, perspective taking, planning, creativity) evolved in the context of solving physical problems. These survival activities were challenges and pursuits that were as much physical as they were mental. Building shelter, navigating terrain, negotiating social situations, escaping from predators, tracking and hunting, creating, and using tools. Compare these activities to those of the typical office worker and it's easy to see how neglecting the body has become the norm.

Advances in technology make life easier. Think of the wonders of cars, telephones, microwaves, and my personal favorite, dishwashers! But this ease comes at the cost of disconnection between our heads and the rest of our bodies. By reducing physical activity to our current sedentary levels, neither our bodies nor brains function optimally.

Brain cells extend throughout our bodies. Our intelligence is a function of our ability to move as embodied beings.

Think about the last time you were in a long staff meeting or sitting for hours. Did your brain feel foggy? Was your body stiff? Moving muscles pump fresh blood and oxygen through the brain and trigger the release of all sorts of brain- and mood-enhancing chemicals. When sitting for prolonged periods of time, every system in the body slows down. including our brains. We can't process information very well or learn as quickly, and problem solving abilities and creativity stagnates.

Because how we work and how we exercise are displaced, we experience a splitting between our minds and our bodies: We have become disembodied minds at work sitting in chairs hunched over keyboards, and mindless bodies at the gym running on treadmills staring at TVs.

When we live with our mind and body disconnected, our actions become incongruent. We go to the gym and feel like that offsets eating the cookies that were left out in the office lunchroom. The different environments with opposing goals compete with our efforts instead of giving us focus and clarity.

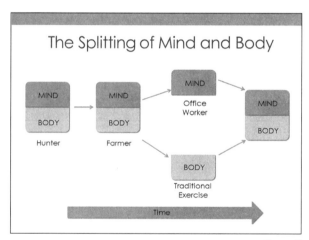

Figure 7

Office Culture versus Traditional Exercise Programs	
Office Culture	**Traditional Exercise Programs**
• Work sitting all day with poor posture • Focus on the activity of the mind only • Encourages workaholics who neglect things like lunch, water, and sleep • There's no time or space for your body at the workplace; take care of your health at the gym if at all • Busy and frantic = productive • Work eight or more hours straight with no breaks • No time for lunch	• Pursue idealized body images based on models, actors and athletes • Train hardcore! If it doesn't hurt, you're not doing it right! • Needs to take place at the gym • Needs a chunk of time out of your day separate from work • Exercising daily or three to four times a week is enough to offset sedentary time (myth)

Figure 8

Unfortunately, actors, models, athletes, fitness instructors, personal trainers, and many others cannot relate to the daily reality of being in an office where everyone sits all day because people in these roles are paid to be physically fit and are moving around constantly. Their physical health has a direct relationship to their work so the connection between exercise and work is meaningful, which makes it easier for them to be motivated to exercise.

For many, traditional exercise programs have no direct or meaningful benefit to their sedentary working lives so it's easy to neglect exercise and prioritize other tasks. The person working in an office may even consider that that hour or two at the gym might be better spent getting work done or having quality time with his or her family.

The hope is not to transform your workplace into something that it is not but to use movement to help optimize what it can be. What could your workplace become if everyone was healthier, free to move, and to take care of their health? What could be accomplished if everyone was more connected to their bodies and had more energy, focus, and joy at work?

This does not mean turning workplaces into gyms — although for some workplaces, this might make sense. Again with a focus on movement not exercise, it means moving so that we are taking care of our backs, stimulating our hearts and brains, improving digestive health, preventing atrophy, and essentially caring for our bodies so we're not wasting our lives going for treatments for preventable illnesses and injuries, but instead pursuing meaningful work. Leadership needs to give people permission to move and individual employees need to give themselves permission to move.

Different forms of movement can be used to stimulate different brain states. This will vary between individuals. For example, imagine you are feeling tired and sluggish. You might do a cardio-based movement in order to get the blood pumping throughout your entire body and to feel re-energized. If you are feeling stressed and overwhelmed by multiple demands, you might use a body awareness practice to help calm your nervous system and move into a more focused and relaxed state. If you are feeling tense and stiff in your chair you could use a flexibility move to loosen the body and reduce tension.

Rather than segregating movement to an hour a day in a location separate from your workplace, why not feed yourself with nutritious movement breaks throughout the day? Moving in this way, you can begin to make the direct connection between your body and working better by experiencing immediate benefits to your productivity. Movement can address the sedentary issue and transform the way you work in the here and now with greater energy, focus, and joy.

In order to evaluate whether what we are doing is best for our health, we need to evaluate health and wellness programs based on their ability to account for the larger and more realistic picture of how we live and work. Does it address the sedentary life we currently live? Is it sustainable in terms of demands of time, money, and energy? Is it work-enhancing or work interfering?

How can we shift our thinking, behavior, and culture so that we can be fit and healthy? What kind of culture would need to be in place for people to move more at the office? What kind of policies would need to be in place? What kind of attitudes would people need to have? What kind of resources would be needed and how would the environment be different? Here is a list of some ideas. Try to think of what would be needed at your workplace.

A new and healthier culture would encompass:

- An open and accepting attitude towards people listening to their bodies and taking care of themselves at work
- Appreciating the mind and body as one whole
- Freedom of employees to do what they need to do to take care of their bodies as long as it does not interfere with their work
- Permission and encouragement from leadership for people to mind their bodies
- People working with freedom to move their bodies and change positions naturally and creatively according to their needs
- Physical spaces in the office that invite and encourage movement (e.g., specific open spaces for movement, a walking circle, a lunging hallway)
- Office furniture that invites many movement possibilities (e.g., sit/stand desks, some fitness equipment)
- Education about the sedentary issue
- Valuing health over body image
- Specific movements that can be integrated in the workplace

- Support to the staff to implement movement and overcome physical and mental barriers

- Both intrinsic and extrinsic rewards for movement and being mindful of health

- Valuing health as the foundation for our work/lives rather than a luxury

- Having systems in place to make movement at work safe, fun, social, and successful

6. A Vision for a New Work Culture

Imagine a future where people go to work fully embodied with their heads attached to a healthy, vibrant body, feeling energized to do great work. Think how wonderful it would be to not have to worry about having to sit all day and instead having the freedom to move. Together, we can make this vision a reality.

Many innovative thinkers including Steve Jobs and Charles Darwin were aware of the negative impact of sitting. They enjoyed going for long walks either to help stimulate their thinking or for having meetings with others. Darwin felt that sitting in his office made his thinking stagnant. He incorporated walks into his schedule twice a day.

7. Moving towards a Healthy Future

We want to have it all: great career, friends and life partner, recreation, good physical and mental health. If we are to actualize these things, we need a different approach for how we integrate these important areas of life. The messages we hear focus solely on deficiencies:

- "If you want a healthier body, get to the gym!"

- "All you have to do is try harder."

- "Just get up earlier and work out."

- "Don't be so lazy!"

These messages are judgmental, unsustainable, and not based in science or reality. If we are going to value and prioritize health, we can't relegate attention to our bodies to one hour a day and then neglect it the rest of the day by locking ourselves up at chairs and desks.

Proper maintenance and care of our health and bodies requires attention daily as well as intermittently throughout the day. In order to meet our physiological and psychological needs and address the sedentary issue, we need to reimagine the way we work and live and change our culture. We can't just be bodies at the gym, mindlessly lifting weights and running on treadmills, then disembodied heads hunched over computers at a desk all day.

Corporations and organizations where employees sit all day can benefit significantly by evolving their ideas of what it means to be profitable and by recognizing the value of health and our bodies in the workplace. Employees working with only their minds at the expense of their bodies will inevitably experience negative consequences for their physical and mental well-being. This ends up costing everyone in the end through illness, injury, absenteeism, loss of productivity, decreased job satisfaction, mental illness, and increased healthcare costs.

My hope as you read this book is to introduce you a new model of health and exercise; one that removes guilt and blame from the individual and makes taking care of your health both an individual and collective pursuit. I hope you will be inspired to transform the culture at least on a local level through your own awareness, perceptions, beliefs, actions, and interactions with others. Most importantly, I hope these ideas have inspired you to think differently about your body and how important your health is.

Face the reality of your work/life context and focus on health rather than on idealized body images or other fantasies of health. I encourage you to become an active participant in your health journey and to see every moment as an opportunity to move towards health.

The ThinkMOVE program is designed to provide both immediate and long term benefits for the person struggling with sitting too much. A person who begins to move more throughout the day will experience the immediate benefits of increased energy, focus, and mood and over the longer term prevent illness, achieve a healthy weight, improve fitness, and prevent premature death.

Change is rarely easy. However, a movement-based approach is accessible for all regardless of age or physical ability. Incorporating movement into your day can be as bite-sized as taking a minute to stand or jogging on the spot for 20 seconds. Normalizing movement at the workplace may seem a bit strange now, but everything new feels strange in the beginning. By seeing health as an individual and collective endeavor that supports the goals of both, we can begin to move organizations towards a new way of working. I hope that the content in this book will make the transition and integration of these ideas as easy as possible.

The ThinkMOVE program is a movement platform that provides support and accountability to empower people to define health and wellness goals on their terms and to take action in meaningful ways that fit within their everyday lives.

8. Cultural Transformations Experienced through ThinkMOVE (or, Testimonials for Starting Your Own Program)

- "I personally had more energy on days that I did ThinkMOVE. Because I was allowed to do stuff for my body throughout the day, I was willing to do more for the organization. Working an extra hour was OK."

- "The morale in the office allowed people to get to know each other more and have fun. It's typically hard to make friends across the hierarchy and it's hard to have fun at work, but with the ThinkMOVE program there was more laughter and more energy in the office."

- "I enjoyed seeing the team do the program on Fridays. We were able to enjoy physical activity. At this time, we were appreciating the corporate cultural acceptance of taking care of the body."

- "ThinkMOVE helped bridge some of those hierarchical barriers between coordinators and managers. Everyone was on an even playing field which allowed us to have better relationships."

4

The Science of Healthy Movement: How Moving a Little Can Transform Your Health

We've explored the cultural side of health and the systemic barriers that stand in the way, including an overemphasis on body image, rapid technological advances leading to a more sedentary lifestyle, and opposing messages between how we should work and how we should exercise. Many current exercise programs and tools available use hyperbolic, pseudo-scientific statements not based in real research that claim that faster, longer, more intense exercise is better for all.

The emphasis here is a different approach, moving away from intensive training programs and instead focusing on how to optimize health for a human being who happens to work in an office. The ThinkMOVE approach integrates key findings from a variety of fields including exercise physiology, epidemiology, sedentary research, and kinesiology and is explained in more detail in Chapter 6.

Researchers often write using technical jargon that makes it difficult for the average person to understand how the studies were designed, how they measured change, and what the average person can do with this information. It is not always clear how to apply the findings to our daily lives. For example, you may have read headlines like, "Sit less than three hours, live two years longer." What does that actually mean and what action can we take in our daily lives? How much less should we sit? How can this be possible at work where sitting is the norm?

Understanding the pillars of ThinkMOVE will help you understand the rationale for the six-week program outlined in Chapter 6, and the benefits of practicing this method throughout the rest of your life. For many, this knowledge will help increase motivation and fuel action. For the healthy skeptic, it will help convince them that an intervention so simple, minimal, and requiring little time can really work. Understanding the science will help you navigate new territory as you explore movement in your everyday life, hopefully giving you confidence as you progress and experience the benefits firsthand. Finally, understanding the main principles will help you find your own unique and creative ways to incorporate movement into your day.

1. The Three Pillars of ThinkMOVE

As discussed, prolonged sitting is associated with premature death as well as increased risk for cardiovascular disease, diabetes, and cancer. Logically, if sitting is the problem then moving around all the time must be the solution. Unfortunately, it's more complicated than that but in typical fashion, the health and fitness industry has come up with all kinds of quirky gadgets to solve the problem. Here are just a few:

- Standing desks so you can stand all day

- Treadmills at desks so you can walk all day

- Wearable technologies like Fitbit and Jawbone

- Pilates balls so you can sit and do core exercises all day

- Portable bicycle pedals under desks (to collect dust)

In moderation, some of these could be effective tools. However, the solution to the sitting disease is not in a single piece of equipment or single position. The human body wasn't designed to do any one thing all day but designed to move in all ways. Variety keeps things fresh and fun, including increasing the spaces in which we move. Rather than restricting movement to the gym, we can fulfill a variety of health needs in all of our environments.

The Three Pillars of the ThinkMOVE program are:

1. Informal movement breaks (fidgeting, taking the stairs, walking to water cooler) from sitting can reduce metabolic risk factors and contribute to daily energy expenditure (calories burned).

2. Formal (planned) movement breaks, when done regularly, can reduce metabolic risk factors for long term illnesses like heart disease and diabetes.

3. Short bursts of moderate to high intensity exercise can produce positive improvements in metabolism and fitness including cardiorespiratory capacity and strength, that are comparable to longer form exercise programs.

Let's take a closer look at each one.

To better understand this section, be familiar with these terms:

Glucose is the main type of sugar in the blood and the major source of energy for the body's cells. It comes from the foods we eat or the body can make from other substances. Glucose is carried to the cells through the bloodstream. Several hormones, including insulin, control glucose levels in the blood.

Insulin is a hormone that lowers the level of glucose in the blood. It's made by the beta cells of the pancreas and released into the blood when the glucose level goes up, such as after eating. Insulin helps glucose enter the body's cells, where it can be used for energy or stored for future use.

Insulin resistance occurs when the body doesn't respond as well to the insulin that the pancreas is making and glucose is less able to enter the cells. People who have insulin resistance may or may not develop Type 2 diabetes.

Researchers use measures of glucose and insulin response since they are important cardiometabolic risk markers for heart disease, pre-diabetes and diabetes.

1.1 Pillar 1: Frequent informal breaks from sedentary time reduce health risk

Flowing water never grows stale. So you've got to just keep on moving.

— Bruce Lee

In a study that included 168 adults, researchers monitored how sedentary participants were throughout the day as well as how many breaks they took from sitting. They gave participants accelerometers, which measured movements of all kinds that occurred naturally throughout their day including standing, fidgeting, walking, and taking the stairs. Participants wore them for seven days straight during all waking hours.

The research team hypothesized that regardless of total sitting time, more frequent breaks in sitting time would be associated with healthier metabolic measures.

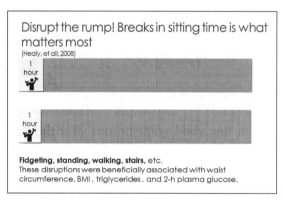

Figure 9

Those who fidgeted, walked around the most, and took the most breaks from sitting had the best health measures according to measurements of blood glucose, abdominal fat, fat content of their blood, and BMI. The positive relationship between breaks of sitting and positive metabolic measures existed even when total sedentary time, exercise time, and intensity of the breaks were accounted for.

They also found that those who took the most breaks from sedentary time had on average 5.95 cm smaller waist circumference than the group with the lowest number of breaks.

This research highlights prolonged sitting as the precursor to health problems, not sitting per se, which means it's not just how much time you sit that matters, it's how that time is accumulated. The detrimental changes in our body composition and metabolism may be due to the absence of muscle contractions which condition our metabolism to slow down because the daily demands for movement are so minimal.

These findings are important because continuous bouts of exercise are not practical for work at the typical office. (No need for a treadmill desk!) Every disruption of sedentary time with movement of any kind adds up to increases of total energy expenditure (calories burned) and helps stoke the fire of our metabolism enough to offset sitting time.

The take home message is: Making short and frequent bouts of movement of any length and intensity can benefit your body as long as they break up sitting time. These frequent informal bits of movement can help you have a thinner waistline, increase your metabolism, and lower the fat content of your blood. Try to keep these benefits in mind as you go about your day and see possibilities for movement: stairs versus escalator, walking over to your coworker versus emailing, getting water, standing, and fidgeting during phone calls and meetings.

Taking a Stand Against Sitting

Dr. Joan Vernikos, a researcher from NASA's life sciences division, discovered that the simple act of standing counteracted the cardiovascular health risks associated with sitting. Her research found that standing up once every hour was more effective than walking on a treadmill for 15 minutes continuously for the regulation of blood pressure and restoration of blood volume after long periods of being sedentary. To her, this makes sense since standing without exercise requires the heart to pump blood up to the head against gravity without the help of contracting leg muscles.

Dr. Vernikos recommends shorter but more frequent changes in posture in order to benefit the regulation of blood pressure. In her book *Sitting Kills, Moving Heals,* (Quill Driver Books, 2011) she writes, "standing up often is what matters, not how long you remain standing." In fact, the longer you stand the less blood vessel walls are stimulated, which is important for healthy blood flow. Keep that in mind for those who have standing desks. Long periods in any sedentary position results in less stimulation of muscles therefore it's best to practice shifting positions and moving frequently throughout the day.

"Every time you stand up, the body initiates a shift in fluids and hormones and causes muscle contraction to occur; and almost every nerve in the body is stimulated. If you stand up 16 times a day for minutes (each time), the body would read that as 16 stimuli, whereas if you stood once for 32 minutes, it would see that as one stimulus."

To get the heart benefits, she recommends standing up 35 times a day which works out to being about once every 20–30 minutes depending on how much you sit. She suggests that the stimulus (standing, moving) must be spread throughout the day.

Have you ever noticed how hungry you feel after a long, intense workout? For anyone who has ever struggled to lose weight despite exercising, researchers are finding that acute bouts of exercise (i.e., traditional methods of exercise) create something called the caloric consumption effect, which is the release of hormones which increase appetite. Researchers are finding that " … unlike bouts of moderate to vigorous activity, low-intensity ambulation, standing, walking around, fidgeting, taking out the garbage may contribute to daily expenditure without triggering the caloric consumption effect." This may be a familiar phenomenon to many who have overeaten after a grueling workout and felt badly afterwards.

1.2 Pillar 2: Frequent BREAKS of formal movement improve metabolism

Most sedentary research consists of observational studies which make it difficult to comment on causation. An intervention study lead by Dr. Dunstan gives some unique insights into the power of regular movement breaks on our metabolism.

The researchers hypothesized that metabolism would improve by brief intermittent bouts of activity, whether these breaks were of light or moderate intensity. The study recruited overweight/obese adults aged 45-65 for a three period, three treatment acute trial:

GROUP 1: Uninterrupted sitting for the five-hour period.

GROUP 2: Seated with two-minute bouts of light-intensity walking every 20 minutes.

GROUP 3: Seated with two-minute bouts of moderate-intensity walking every 20 minutes.

Each treatment condition lasted five hours, resulting in 28 minutes (14 breaks X 2 minutes each) of physical activity spread over the five hours. Everyone had the chance to try all three conditions to create comparisons within and between participants. As in the previous study, participants wore accelerometers to measure activity level.

The results showed that just a few minutes of light walking every 20 minutes improved the body's ability to process glucose by an impressive 24 percent and insulin levels by 23 percent! Both insulin and glucose are important metabolic markers for reducing risk of cardiac disease and Type 2 diabetes.

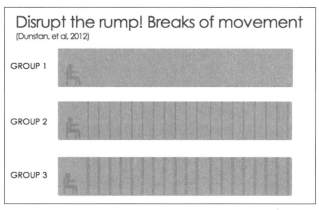

Figure 10

Researchers found that metabolic changes found in the five-hour pure sitting condition (group 1) was similar to studies where people sat for an entire day suggesting that the movement breaks were an effective way to address the effects of sitting. In a conversation with Travis Saunders, a key sedentary researcher, he explained that, "Drug companies would be thrilled to get these results!" These findings also confirm the observational studies that prolonged sitting has negative effects on health and that too much sitting is distinct from too little exercise.

The study suggests that using light intensity movements throughout the day can reduce the risk of cardiovascular disease and diabetes. Interestingly, the results found using brief intermittent bouts of activity (2 minutes of walking every 20 minutes) were comparable to changes in insulin and glucose levels after a single bout of exercise (30 minutes of jogging) found in other studies. A few of the benefits of using intermittent movement breaks over single exercise sessions are: they can be of lower intensity, the time commitment is minimal, and it addresses the problem of sitting all day.

These findings ought to be encouraging for those who either do not enjoy going to the gym or don't have time. Office workers who do not exercise can have confidence in knowing that with short bits of movement spread regularly throughout their day they can achieve similar results as the person who sets aside time for exercise while also addressing the sedentary issue; a two-for-one deal!

How this looks in the ThinkMOVE program:

1. **Movement is prioritized over exercise**: According to the research, movement breaks are capable of achieving similar physiological

benefits as exercise while simultaneously addressing the sedentary issue. This is great news for the average office worker who is part of the 95 percent of people who struggle to fit in enough exercise or even the person who exercises regularly but is sedentary for most of the day. Thinking "MOVE" instead of "I have to get to the gym" is one of most significant mindset shifts to impact your health. By bringing movement into our daily lives in chunks of all shapes and sizes (big, small, high or low intensity, long or short), we can reap the physical and mental health benefits of exercise.

2. **Movement every 20 minutes:** The research reviewed used 20 minutes as the standard period between breaks and 2 minutes for the actual movement breaks. The ThinkMOVE program recommends a similar protocol but you will build up to this. At first you might start off with three simple breaks a day each lasting only one minute scheduled at specific times of the day. As you progress, you will try to move every 20 minutes. Some movements are so simple and easy that you can do them while continuing to work, while others will only require a minute or two away from your work. This minute or two spent moving is designed to help you regain energy and refocus your attention.

1.3 Pillar 3: A little bit of high-intensity movement will help you get fitter and stronger

Hopefully, you are beginning to see that little bits of movement can significantly reduce the negative effects of sitting by improving insulin sensitivity and blood glucose. You might also be wondering, "What's the point of setting aside time to exercise?" It's a good question considering lack of time is often cited as a major barrier to exercise.

Exercising is good for your health because it improves metabolic and cardiovascular functioning, strength, prevents muscle atrophy, helps maintain a healthy weight, and supports mental health. A growing body of research on High Intensity Interval Training (HIIT) is calling into question traditional notions of exercise, particularly the amount of time it should take. If you're someone who wants to know "What is the minimum amount of exercise I can do?", the emerging evidence is showing it might be a lot less than we think.

Exploring alternative methods of exercise is important for people who don't have enough time, interest, or desire to add long bouts of exercise into their day. In a culture where more, faster, longer exercise is the ideal, what you are about to read may feel like cheating or being lazy. I'd invite you to approach this introduction to HIIT as if it were a new technology like Netflix that made video stores obsolete. HIIT will help you train smarter. It will save you time and money and it will help you get healthier. If you enjoy working out and you use it as time to get away and mentally recharge, then I respect the sacredness of that time and space. But for many people, the gym or exercise is not heaven.

HIIT is essentially short bursts of all-out effort (lasting 15–30 seconds), which, in research, has typically been done with sprints on an exercise bike. Research is showing that doing HIIT-style workouts creates physiological changes similar to traditional hour long cardio sessions but in 90 percent less time.

Studies comparing HIIT workouts to traditional endurance training have found no difference between their ability to improve skeletal muscle adaptations, metabolism, and cardio capacity. Incorporating high intensity movement breaks into your day may enable you to gain many of the benefits of exercise.

1.4 What is the least amount of exercise I can do?

In one study from the UK involving 29 sedentary men and women, researchers had participants perform three workouts a week for six weeks totaling 18 sessions. Each session involved only two intense cardio sprints lasting 15–20 seconds each. These sprints took place on a stationary bike. Each session lasted ten minutes with a three-minute warm up, 20-second sprint, three-minute break between sprints, 20-second sprint, and three-minute cool down.

The highest Rating for Perceived Exertion (RPE) (the participants' self rating) was 14 out of 20. That translates to about 75 percent perceived effort, which was well tolerated by all participants, especially when they considered the amount of time they were saving. Other studies have used this type of protocol with cardiac patients. That might seem counterintuitive, but so far no problems have been reported. Dr. Maureen MacDonald, an associate professor of Kinesiology at McMaster University, also looking at the effects of HIIT, said, "It appears that the heart is insulated from the intensity of the intervals because the effort is so brief."

It's important to separate the warm-up and cool-down time from HIIT time because what researchers are suggesting is it is the high levels of glycogen depletion that occurs with short burst of high intensity cardio that regulates insulin sensitivity. Of course, warming up the body is always important.

After six weeks, the study found significant improvement in insulin sensitivity (28 percent improvement) and aerobic capacity (15 percent improvement for men, 12 percent for women). Another study found similar results in only two weeks! Excluding warm-up and cool down, the participants only did nine-and-a-half minute workouts over the course of six weeks. That's an average of a minute-and-a-half of working out per week. If you don't have a 90 seconds per week then you must be the busiest person on the planet.

If I still haven't convinced you of the benefits of short bursts of activity, let me leave you with an analogy to compare these two scenarios: HIIT versus traditional cardio. Imagine something you really want. It could be an object or a goal like better health. Now imagine you had to travel by foot to get to the exact same goal and you are given two choices: you could choose to jog steadily for 150 minutes for a distance of 28,000 meters (91,863.5 feet), or you could sprint for 20 seconds, six times (two minutes total) spaced with light walking in between for a total of 700 meters (2,296.5 feet).

The average human jogs at 11 km (6.84 miles) per hour. In 150 minutes that would be a distance of 28 km. The average human sprints at 21 km (13 miles) per hour. In two minutes, that would be a distance of about 700 meters. Fun fact: in the same time, Usain Bolt, who can run 45 km/h (28 mph) would travel 1,200 meters!

Which one of these would you choose? Which one of these do you have time and energy for? These time and distance differences are comparable when comparing HIIT workouts to traditional endurance training. With HIIT, you not only save the time but also the wear and tear on the body's joints and ligaments.

If you enjoy running as a sport and find it rewarding, that's great. For those who don't think exercise and fun belong in the same sentence, short bouts of high intensity training can improve health with minimal time expenditure.

We have applied these research concepts into our program and observed significant changes in people's fitness levels. Before we begin our program, everyone performs a fitness assessment which measures strength, core strength, balance, and cardio. Here is a breakdown of each test:

- **Strength test (push ups):** This would be the total number of push ups a person can do in two minutes. These push ups can be standard with knees up, knees down, or against the wall. There can be breaks in between repetitions.

- **Core strength test (plank):** Get into the position displayed and hold for as long as possible. Be mindful of keeping a neutral spine.

- **Balance test (Standing Superman):** Take turns standing on one foot. The idea is to hold your hands out in front of you and one leg behind you creating a flat surface. Stretch as far as you can and hold the position for as long as possible.

- **Cardio test (squats):** Try doing rapid squats at a pace of one squat per second to engage the cardiovascular system. The test is over when you can no longer keep the one squat per second pace and you need to take a break. What usually happens is the lactic acid builds up and the individual needs to stop.

After doing our introductory program, participants in MOVE averaged six-and-a-half MOVE breaks per day, which took only about ten minutes spread throughout the day, over nine weeks with a variety of exercises. Results are shown in Figure 11.

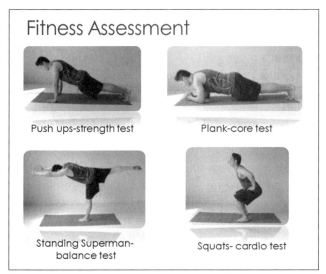

Figure 11

Impressively, every measure of fitness improved significantly. The group's strength improved by 26 percent, core strength by 61 percent, balance by 36 percent, and cardio by 103 percent. We did not have the ability to measure insulin sensitivity or glucose, but the largest improvement was found in the cardio test at 103 percent, which is aligned with improvements in aerobic capacity found in the studies we've discussed. Unlike the HIIT studies, participants in the Think-MOVE program were doing cardio breaks at perceived exertion of low to moderate levels, which suggests that every bit of effort counts, even if it's not a full-out sprint or at maximum intensity.

2. How All of This Looks in ThinkMOVE

2.1 ThinkMOVE method incorporates HIIT

As you become more comfortable with moving periodically through-out the day, try adding higher intensity move breaks. Doing HIIT-style MOVE breaks will depend on your personal level of fitness and your current work culture. If you're not comfortable doing this style of move-ment at work, you could begin to try doing a few bursts of cardio in the evening when you're at home watching Netflix. For example, you could do light jogging on the spot for 40–45 seconds and then go all out for the last 15–20 seconds. Always give your body a chance to warm up and get used to the movement before increasing the intensity.

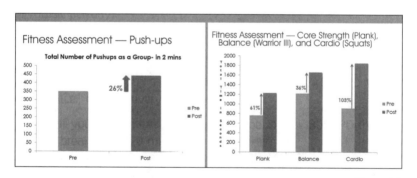

Figure 12

If you walk regularly, you might incorporate a couple of sprints to ignite your metabolism and challenge your fitness. Doing high intensity cardio moves before meals will increase your metabolism for that meal.

If you walk regularly for your daily commute, jogging might not be feasible due to dress or bags you need to carry, but you could try walking as fast as you can for 20 seconds and then at normal speed for a minute, and repeating that a few times.

There are many ways to apply HIIT into your life. Just think short, intense bursts, lasting 20–30 seconds, and experiment with when and where this could fit in your life. For some, walking or sprinting up the stairs would be high intensity.

2.2 Cardio breaks

Try cardio breaks right from the beginning if possible. Although our initial focus is on improving overall body awareness and flexibility, incorporate a few cardio moves every other day lasting a minute each time. You'll likely find your energy levels going way up as well as your ability to concentrate throughout the day. Generally if you want to incorporate more cardio into your week, you could start with three to four cardio MOVEs every other day and that would give you either 9 or 12 sprints a week, which is more than what was done in the UK study.

3. Variety Is the Spice of Life

Just as sitting all day is not healthy, neither is standing or walking all day. Thankfully, technological advances have given us the option to choose how we use (or don't use) our bodies. This research challenges traditional ways to approach health and exercise as well as previous time prescriptions for exercise (e.g., the 150 minutes of activity).

Given the fact that 95 percent of people are not able to fit the standard physical activity guidelines into their lives, it's time to think outside the box. The research points to new and exciting possibilities. Essentially, we can address the sedentary issue by disrupting periods of sitting with movement and we can integrate bits of exercise in formal but conveniently short bouts.

The body needs variety: varieties of movement and varieties of intensity (light, moderate, and vigorous). The ThinkMOVE program provides variety by including five categories of movement: strength, cardio, core/balance, flexibility, and the foundational skill of body awareness. By integrating these practices into your day and at various times throughout the day, you will be able to work on areas of health that you might never have spent time on before.

In the next chapter, we will explore the process of changing a sedentary culture to a movement-based culture and how to overcome natural resistances to change both internally and externally.

Prolong Your Life by 22 Minutes with Just 3 Minutes

Research from Australia found that every hour of television watched (taken as a measure of sitting time) after the age of 25 reduces the person's life expectancy by 22 minutes.

Other research suggests that if people sit three hours or less a day they can expect to live two years longer! Life expectancy is a population statistic and it does not apply to specific individuals. It is logical that breaking up sitting time will also increase life expectancy, which is why I recommend taking a MOVE break once every 20 minutes.

Increasing Life Expectancy Calculation: (Just for Fun!)

Our general guideline is to do a 1-minute MOVE break every 20 minutes. That means for every hour of sitting time there will be three breaks from sitting totaling 3 minutes. Given our discussion of the research and the physiological improvements, it is hoped this intervention successfully addresses the sedentary issue which in turn prolongs your life. Further long-term studies need to be done to validate this hypothesis. It's not hard to believe that moving more and using the five categories will help improve the quality of your life by strengthening muscles and bones, strengthening your heart, improving flexibility and range of motion, as well as your ability to balance and go up stairs. For now, you can think that your return on time investment for doing 3 minutes of movement every hour is prolonging your life by 22 minutes or approximately 7 minutes for every minute of MOVE you do.

These numbers aren't to be taken literally but as a way to get you thinking about the concrete value that moving more can have in terms of prolonging life expectancy and reversing the effects of being sedentary.

If you calculate 7 minutes for every minute of MOVE done, the calculation would work like this: Sally does nine MOVE breaks over the course of three hours. (9 X 7 = 63) She may have extended her life expectancy by 63 minutes!

Exercise 4
Motivating towards Movement: Reflection Questions and Experiments

These questions and experiments will help you anchor your learning and begin practicing moving more throughout your day. Reflect on any new awareness you may have as a result of reading these chapters and consider what you are willing to change in your life.

1. Considering how many hours you sit per day, how does sitting make you feel? Are you willing to incorporate movement breaks into your day? What changes would you hope to experience? What would need to happen for you to be successful with this?

2. Reflect on your own workplace. How open would your coworkers and managers be if you were to begin to incorporate movement into your day? Try inviting a coworker to do a stretch break with you or to go for a walking meeting.

3. If you are someone who does not enjoy exercise, how has the information in this last chapter impacted the way you see yourself and exercise? Are you willing to incorporate more movement and perhaps higher intensity movement breaks into your day? Try doing at least one cardio move every other day this week and see how it makes you feel.

5

The Process of Change and Overcoming Resistance to Movement

The previous chapters have hopefully shed some light on the problem of sitting as well as how it can be addressed by periodic bouts of movement. Despite the scientific evidence, I imagine the idea of moving at the workplace is still challenging for many. Perhaps some of these thoughts have occurred as you've been reading:

- "This is great in theory, but I'll look silly exercising at work."

- "People will judge me."

- "I can't move in these clothes."

- "I'm too busy!"

- "It doesn't look professional. What if our clients see us moving?"

These are all forms of "Yes, but ... ," which are natural forms of resistance familiar to anyone who's ever tried to make a health change. Along the path of growth and change, the voice of resistance will surely rear its fearful head. It is important to become aware of resistance and address each concern in turn. It is a natural human instinct to fear and resist change. Change can be scary because it is unknown and we can't always be sure how it will impact our lives. For example, how will making a health change impact relationships, or how much free time I have? Resistance can often bring up legitimate concerns.

In this chapter, we explore the top resistances to movement and address each with suggestions related to mindset as well as practical techniques and actions. It is up to the individual to determine whether he or she is challenged by a legitimate barrier or is simply using excuses that get in the way.

When it comes to making meaningful and powerful health changes, like those of ThinkMOVE, I don't know if it's ever possible to avoid having to face challenges and resistance. The person and organization that is willing to face the resistance head-on and in an honest way will be successful. It comes down to the choices the individual and organization make to prioritize health and to make movement possible.

ThinkMOVE is the practice of making healthy choices daily. Most people aren't aware of how much choice they have to get out of old unhealthy habits, including the sitting habit. The freedom to choose exists in our ability to choose our attitudes, behavior, and priorities.

I'll give you a small example of a health behavior change that illustrates overcoming resistance. As I write this, my wife, Le Le, is seven months pregnant. She takes the train into work. Because we live in Toronto, there is rarely a seat available for her. As she started to show and she gained weight, she became concerned that she would fall while standing on the train.

She would come home every day complaining that no one would freely offer her a seat and worried that she would one day fall or be bumped. I was quite concerned knowing how crowded the trains can be during rush hour. I encouraged her to ask people sitting in priority seating designated for disabled, pregnant, and elderly passengers to give up their seats. She resisted this for weeks because she feared confrontation or being ignored by others, but as her belly grew so did her resolve. Eventually, her anger at the insensitive and mindless rush hour passengers moved her to make her request for a seat. In this scenario, making the request for a seat is a healthy behavior.

In order to make this change, Le Le had to prioritize her health and the health of our baby. It may seem like such a small behavior, but because of the stress of a packed train, she needed to gather her resolve to ask for someone's seat daily. I'm so proud of her!

Prioritizing and committing to health have similar factors at play when it comes to incorporating healthy movement during the day. Changing the sitting habit alone is very difficult when a person works in a sedentary environment, therefore creating teams and social connection through the program is important.

Change always feels strange in the beginning. It can feel awkward to even imagine moving at the office. This is why I was so resistant to doing my rehab exercises in the first place. I didn't think it was professional or appropriate to exercise at the office. It wasn't until the pain was so bad and persistent that I gave up caring about others' judgments of me and moved so that I could feel healthy again. Over time, people started to ask me what I was up to, and I shared what I was learning. It became a fun activity for all of us to do at the office.

We have all been taught to sit still and be quiet; to ignore the body unless it is dirty, sick, or in pain. The idea of listening, attending, and caring for our bodies throughout the day is challenging to the status quo. It's natural that anyone considering making a health change like ThinkMOVE will face internal and external resistance.

1. The Top Ten Resistances to Movement at the Office and How to Overcome Them

There are ten main resistances you may encounter when beginning to implement movement into your day. All ten barriers can occur at any stage of change; however, some of these experiences are more likely to occur at earlier stages, such as past failures, which may impede one's willingness to consider trying something new. Other factors occur at later stages of change. For example, a lack of permission from the organization's leadership team may be a barrier to those who are highly motivated to act, but are concerned about being judged.

1. **Self-conscious thoughts:** "I'm going to look dumb." "People will judge me." The feelings that underlie these thoughts are fear of being judged or standing out from the crowd. People may feel self-conscious about their ability to move well, "What if I do the exercises incorrectly and look stupid?," or "I prefer to move privately because I don't want people looking at my body." This barrier sometimes relates to a person's feelings of low self-worth and negative perceptions of his or her body that make it difficult to imagine successful outcomes.

   Overcoming self-conscious thoughts requires self-acceptance and letting go of trying to meet others' expectations. You might think, "Others may judge me, but I own my health and

I own my decision to move. I accept myself and let go of the need for everyone else's approval."

2. **Past failures with health programs and low confidence that anything will help:** "I've tried so many exercise programs and fad diets in the past and they haven't worked. How will ThinkMOVE be different?" ThinkMOVE is designed to be a low time-demand program that is integrated into the work day.

3. **Work pressures (time pressure) and feeling under the gun:** "I have so much to do … I am afraid that looking away from my work for even for a minute will take me off course." Leaders of organizations are especially vulnerable to this pattern since they feel they need to set the tone for the rest of the organization by working hard and working long hours. The pace and intensity of work depend greatly on the overall work culture.

   You can deal with this by talking with your boss and colleagues. Let them know that you want to take these brief one minute movement breaks to reset your body and mind so you can take care of your health and work better. The practice itself will address any further concerns because you will be more productive and energized.

4. **Others' actual judgments in the form of criticism or teasing:** People may think it's funny to put down others trying to take care of their health at work. I've witnessed people commenting on people's diet choices all the time at work and it can feel embarrassing to put yourself out there in public as someone trying to do something healthy. Because most offices are unhealthy, this is seen as deviant behavior and draws attention which is sometimes negative. Similarly to Resistance #1, it's important to not internalize other people's judgments. Often, people's reactions have to do with their own insecurities or health struggles. Focus on yourself and why taking care of your health is important for you. Share what you are doing with those who seem open and build a community of movers around you.

5. **Performance anxiety:** "What if I try and I don't do as much as others?" "What if I don't meet my own or others' expectations?" "I haven't done it in a while and I feel resistance to starting up again." It's quite common that people's ambitions to do things well or perfectly get in the way of them engaging in the program. To reduce performance anxiety, it is important

to relax and use ThinkMOVE as a way of coping with stress rather than allowing it to become a source of stress. Do your best and accept that your best is good enough.

6. **Low motivation:** "I just don't care enough to do anything about this." Because of the low time-demand of ThinkMOVE, people can try it without needing a high level of motivation. Experiencing the early benefits of moving more will likely increase motivation.

7. **Management:** The culture at your work may not permit movement at the office. Upper management may perceive a program like ThinkMOVE to be unnecessary since people should just be working and not be concerned with health at the workplace. Support from management is critical as it sets the tone for the work culture. Starting the conversation and sharing the potential benefits of movement is a good place to start. If they are still resistant, there are many ways to incorporate movement that don't require approval, such as the exercises in this book that can be done from a seated position.

8. **Lack of physical space:** Offices come in all sizes and shapes. Some environments have desks crammed together and offer little privacy or space to move one's body. Many exercises in this book require little space like mountain bends (explained later), squats, the neck/wrist routine, and the hamstring/glute stretches. Choose the exercises that you can do and try not to worry about what you can't do. Perhaps you can step into an empty meeting room and do your MOVE break there if more space is needed. Be creative and don't limit what your body can do based on external circumstances.

9. **Wardrobe limitations:** "I wear skirts/dresses/high heels a lot and I worry that moving is going to be difficult and uncomfortable." Many outfits worn in a business setting are not conducive to movement. This is another factor that contributes to the overall pattern of sedentary behavior at work. Like lack of physical space, focus on the moves you can do and perhaps wear more flexible clothes a few days a week so you can practice strength and cardio moves. At the very least standing up, walking, and stretching once every 20–40 minutes will help you address sedentary time and improve your energy and focus.

10. **Accountability and support**: "What am I supposed to do exactly?" "How am I supposed to do it?" "When and where can I do it?" "How will I keep track of my efforts so I can see and measure progress and know what I am doing well and where I need to improve?" "I need encouragement and support to do things for my health and to move." The ThinkMOVE program was created with accountability and support in mind. The information in this book is your guide to answering the what, when, where, why, and how of moving at work.

2. The Satir Change Model

Virginia Satir, a pioneer of family therapy, developed a model of how individuals and families experience change. The Satir Change Model explains that, as we experience significant change, we move through stages: Status Quo, Foreign Element, Chaos, Transforming Idea, Practice and Integration, and New Status Quo (see Figure 13). In the case of ThinkMOVE, both the individual and the organization are changing their behavior so the individual is incorporating healthy bouts of movement throughout the day and the organization is accepting and supporting this. As we have discussed, resistance is an inevitable part of the change process. We will discuss what the experience might look and feel like at both levels so you can be prepared to address any concerns regarding the ThinkMOVE program.

First let's discuss resistance. It is helpful to try to understand what resistance's intentions are for our lives and organization. We have a natural immunity to change because it can invite stress, fear, pain, work, and possible failure, which makes it risky to commit to change.

It's not only failure people avoid. Success comes with a price tag too. Success means exertion of time, energy, and resources, which can be tiring in the face of everything else we have to do. It is important that we don't just frame resistance negatively, as the bad guy. Actually, resistance is like a protective pet that growls at strangers or new experiences. His intention is our well-being and safety. Ironically, resistance, which stems from fear, can leave us stuck in patterns that are no longer useful for us and actually do us harm.

In my work in psychotherapy, I help people approach their resistance in a friendly, compassionate way. We educate the client's resistance to the positive possibilities of change while also listening to its fears. Being respectful and firm with resistance allows it to lower its guard and take in new information.

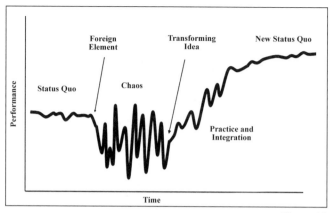

Figure 13

2.1 Status quo

Status quo is what is known and familiar. This is where we feel most comfortable and represent our learned habits.

When it comes to physical movement in an office environment, individual employees and the entire company have established behavioral patterns of working in a sedentary routine. As sedentary time accumulates, health (both physical and mental) begins to worsen as a result of excessive sitting, and companies can expect employee performance declines as a result. However, the decline is gradual and goes unnoticed at first.

Eventually, employees become better at ignoring their bodies and feeling disconnected from their bodies. Some people may experience the pain of being stiff and sore from sitting. They may have also noticed incremental weight gain or decreased energy, but for the most part they are not yet motivated to do anything about it. Noticing these symptoms of health decline becomes familiar and normalized as coworkers share similar experiences of back pain and weight gain, though they might not be aware of a way to change things. Sitting for prolonged periods of time is status quo in the office environment.

People at this stage are said to be precontemplative (Prochaska, 1983), which means they are mostly uninformed and unmotivated to change their behavior.

None of the ten resistances to movement has come up because no change has been introduced to the person or company yet. If you've read this far into the book, you are no longer precontemplative.

2.2 The foreign element

The foreign element is the event, person, idea, or program that helps identify the limits of the status quo. In the context of the sedentary problem, the foreign element is the idea that sitting is the root of many health issues and movement throughout the day can transform your health positively. Hopefully, the information in this book has helped transform some of your assumptions about health and fitness. For example, sitting has negative effects on your health whether you exercise or not.

This new awareness is a foreign element. It is foreign because it comes from outside of your world of sitting. It challenges your assumptions and offers new hope and possibilities. The ThinkMOVE program aims to be challenging and yet realistic by beginning with moderate changes. The program introduced in later chapters introduces only a few simple MOVE breaks lasting a minute each. It builds up from there until the MOVE habit becomes integrated seamlessly.

Through the process of change, it is beneficial to practice appreciating yourself for your willingness to improve your health and embrace change. Notice the early changes you make and celebrate them. These little changes form the foundation for larger, lasting changes.

People at this stage are contemplative; they are still on the fence. They are open to ideas about changing their behavior, but have not made a decision or a commitment to change. They are considering the pros and cons of changing and exploring their choices.

The resistances that people are likely grappling with at this stage include low motivation, self-conscious thoughts, and low confidence from past failures. These resistances make it difficult to imagine success. Having a clear and compelling goal for your health will help you build motivation.

As for self-conscious thoughts, having a compelling reason is a powerful way to overcome negative judgments; your own or others'. For you, it might be wanting to be there for your loved ones, or reaching your retirement with a healthy body so you can enjoy life. Finally, connecting with colleagues who will support and move with you is another way to overcome self-conscious thoughts.

2.3 Chaos

At first these new ideas about health, movement, and the sitting disease may put you in a state of chaos, where you realize what you've been doing isn't working anymore and you are open to exploring change.

The chaos period involves creating new awareness as well as contemplating and preparing for change. Overall this is the most active period of the change process because you are building up your willingness to change and exploring what choices are available.

New awareness brings you into unfamiliar territory. Having read this far, it may be clearer to you why adopting a regular exercise program has been difficult or why in spite of eating well and exercising you feel tired and sluggish after a day of sitting.

This state of new awareness and contemplating change can feel scary, which may fuel resistance to change. You might be tempted to remain in status quo because it feels stable and familiar there.

During the chaos phase, people need a lot of support to progress through the stages make a decision to move for their health. They may be very serious about joining the program or trying ThinkMOVE at work, but are afraid of being judged or laughed at. It is important now to gather a network of support. This may include family, friends and coworkers who will encourage and keep you accountable.

Inevitably this stage will create some stress as it is unfamiliar. With lots of new information, you may feel that you need to remember and do everything perfectly. As you begin to learn the skills and try to establish the habit, you may miss moving as much as you would like from one day to the next or you may struggle to master MOVE skills. Remind yourself that this is normal. Learn from your reactions.

Giving and receiving support is an important part of making it through the chaos stage. Let others know you are wanting to do the ThinkMOVE program and are worried about being judged or perceived negatively. Ask if they will support you by joining you or at least reserving judgment. For those doing the program with a team, talk to others about any struggles you may have and what you need. Listen to what is going on and offer support. As a community, share creative solutions to overcoming resistances. Reach out to your MOVE team or others who might be interested in ThinkMOVE who can support and keep you on target with your goals.

2.4 Transforming idea

After contemplating change and building willpower, a decision to change or not change is made. The transforming idea is to MOVE. This commitment needs to made repeatedly. The previous stages helped bring you to the point of deciding to prioritize your health and to move. Perhaps you have already decided that your health matters and that you will no longer sacrifice it to please others.

I have provided a large body of reasons, research, and analysis as to why one should MOVE, but the only way to know whether this transforming decision will improve your health is by putting it into action and experiencing the benefits when you move. Fundamentally, Think-MOVE is about moving and improving all of you, not just your body but your mind, your attitude, confidence, connections, work, and vitality.

2.5 Practice and integration

In the practice and integration stage, you start to implement the ideas of MOVE by practicing disrupting sitting time with movement. Each week in the ThinkMOVE program, you will learn new ways to trigger movement in your day as well as new movements in the five categories: body awareness, flexibility, balance, strength, and cardio.

The more you practice, the faster you will learn the exercises and the MOVE skills. Early on, you will experience health benefits in the form of increased energy and mood, improved fitness, increased productivity, and greater social connections at work. Your progress might slip every now and then, but try to take these moments as opportunities for learning what gets in the way and what you need to overcome resistance.

Movement is accessible at any moment of the day. This means that you can create a way of moving that fits you, your personality and your life. Different from formal exercise, you will sense that you are moving towards something new, exciting, and limitless. You may notice your performance improving at your job because you have more energy that may also translate to more time and energy for your home life.

Try not to think of off-days as failures. They offer feedback about what you need. I heard a martial arts coach say, "We win or we learn." The learning frame is constructive in trying to build the moving habit.

Work pressure is a common resistance that comes up during the practice phase. A marketing director told me about a day when she wasn't able to get in even one move break. "I was so busy, people were calling me, coming to my desk. I couldn't breathe." She felt badly for missing her MOVEs, but she remembered to have compassion for herself. This enabled her to think of simple ways she could incorporate movement by simply standing and stretching at her desk while she talked on the phone or suggesting that her coworkers walk and talk with her for a few minutes as they moved in the hallways between meetings. Compassion created the space needed for her to create solutions.

Progress can be measured by the number of MOVEs you do, your consistency, and the level of challenge of movements you do. Those with Type A, high-achieving personalites, may put pressure on themselves to do well with their ThinkMOVE programs. Be aware of thoughts of what you have to, or ought to do as this pattern may become the resistance that interferes with taking MOVE breaks. To overcome resistance to movement, it is more important that you face the reality of your situation rather than focus solely on what you should do.

Every experience you have, whether you are moving or sedentary, contains information for you, which can be a learning opportunity. When you find yourself struggling to incorporate MOVE in your day, let yourself pause and become aware of what is happening. Then try to strategize and adjust what you are doing.

Rather than simply saying, "I'm too busy" and quitting, take a moment to comprehend your situation and think about what you would be willing to do in that moment. Perhaps you can take a MOVE break 15 minutes from now, or perhaps you can stand briefly while you continue to work. In-the-moment strategizing, planning, and adjustments are a part of the process, especially in the beginning.

Acceptance of the natural waves of struggle and resistance is an important part of the process of learning to move throughout the day.

Try to MOVE in as many different situations and times of the day as possible. In this program explained in Chapter 6, each week one of the five categories of ThinkMOVE is introduced. Find out what MOVEs work for you and which ones do not. Allow yourself to play and experiment with the tools and exercises in the program.

It is important that your workplace is a safe environment to practice movement. Encourage your peers to try a MOVE break with you. Let them know what you are up to and that it would be helpful if they could be positive or if they could at least reserve judgments and teasing. It only takes a minute!

As you go through this stage of practice, remember to appreciate yourself for trying something new, taking risks, and learning.

2.6 The new status quo

Your ability to incorporate the ThinkMOVE approach begins to stabilize as you master your MOVE skills. You continue to experience benefits while requiring less effort and attention. Because you are taking care of your health, you can turn your attention to other important areas of your life with more energy, strength, flexibility, self-awareness, control, knowledge, and confidence. Eventually, your MOVE skills become second nature, and your learning becomes new patterns at work. With health as the foundation for your work, your performance can reach new heights and a new status quo is formed.

Progress in the ThinkMOVE program is measured and recognized by advancing through various levels. These levels are a guideline that participants can use to challenge themselves to grow in the program. Using a similar structure as a martial arts belt system, the ThinkMOVE system can be divided into six major levels of progress. See Figure 14. If this motivates you, use it.

Stages of MOVE

White Belt (weeks 1–3)	Green Belt (3–6 months)
• Averaging 3 breaks a day • Feeling self-conscious, weird, guilty about MOVEing at work • Starting to notice discomfort with prolonged sitting TOTAL MOVES: 63	• Averaging 9 to 10 breaks a day • Increased awareness of body; can initiate breaks without alarm; self-promoting • It feels uncomfortable to sit for long periods of time and awareness of discomfort occurs more frequently TOTAL MOVES: 1,119
Yellow Belt (weeks 4–6)	Brown Belt (6–12 months)
• Averaging 5 to 6 breaks a day • Feeling less self-conscious • Feeling energized/focused TOTAL MOVES: 189	• Averaging 11 to 14 MOVES a day • Doing MOVE breaks has become a natural part of your day TOTAL MOVES: 3,551
Blue Belt (weeks 7–9)	Black Belt (12 months +)
• Averaging 7 to 8 breaks a day • Some challenges maintaining gains • Confident in addressing sedentary time • Better food choice, less guilt about not working out at the gym TOTAL MOVES: 359	• Averaging 15+ MOVES a day • Being sedentary feels like a choice • Don't need a timer • Sedentary time is maximum 2 to 3 hours a day • Have mastered a variety of MOVES TOTAL MOVES: 6,071

Figure 14

3. Ten Powerful Choices to get you MOVE-ing!

Absorb what is useful, reject what is useless, and add what is essentially your own.

— Bruce Lee

We will address each of the ten resistances to movement by reviewing ten choices that represent both mindset shifts and actions that can be taken to address barriers to movement. It is important that through practicing movement people become better at making choices about their body and health.

Through the practice of ThinkMOVE, people become more connected to their bodies including feelings, physical sensations, breath, tensions, and they can make healthier choices of how to cope with their experience. The ThinkMOVE program helps people become more accepting and caring towards themselves and as a result people start to develop a more positive relationship with themselves and their bodies.

Here are ten empowering choices you can use to support your movement practice. Keep Bruce Lee's wise words in mind as you choose what fits, ignore what does not, and create what is essentially your own, in the following sections.

3.1 Choose YOU by prioritizing yourself and your health

Own the decision to be healthy and to move to take care of your health. Making this choice enables you to be at your best on the way to creating the life you truly desire. I wish to help you build a strong foundation of health so you can accomplish and serve the causes and people who matter most to you.

This choice is important for overcoming the resistance of other people's judgments and one's self-consciousness. By making the choice to move and practicing movement, you can move past judgment and negativity by experiencing the benefits of movement.

3.2 Choose to MOVE wherever, whatever, whenever (health integration)

You can always do something good for your body. It can be as simple as standing up and taking a break from sitting for 20 seconds. The ThinkMOVE program focuses on removing barriers to health. We know that the body thirsts for movement and with MOVE, you can feed it anytime. ThinkMOVE can be integrated into your day and takes into account the realities of your time, work demands, and family life.

Choosing to move creatively and flexibly means being committed to overcoming resistances like limits of physical space, restrictive wardrobes, or lack of support from managers. Choosing to MOVE could mean sitting in a meeting and choosing to contract your abs or thigh muscles for 30 seconds to increase blood flow. No one has to know and you would have done something good for your body. Over time your resolve will increase and you will become a champion for movement and not care what people think. Whatever situation you find yourself in, if there is a desire by your body to move, there will be a way to move. Others will be inspired by your example and join you.

3.3 Choose to create balance

ThinkMOVE encourages balance and moderation of all kinds. This includes enjoying food as well as sedentary time. We are not suggesting that you move around all day. We hope to empower people to choose when to sit and when to move rather than being sedentary out of habit or because of their work culture. ThinkMOVE provides the tools and exercises to help people enjoy moments of indulgence while creating healthy habits that occur a majority of the time.

There is often the pressure to work in a rushed and pressured rhythm to meet deadlines. Following everyone else's rhythm and saying yes to every project is a recipe for burnout and disease. It's fine to work quickly when the situation demands. But it is also important to use MOVE breaks as an anchor to stay connected to yourself throughout your day. This will help you gain energy and maintain balance. Taking 30 seconds to a minute to move and stretch once every 20–30 minutes will not interfere with your work productivity. In fact, it will help you maintain a high work output.

3.4 Choose to be resilient and start again

ThinkMOVE makes it easier to bounce back from missed workouts, long periods of sitting, or unhealthy food choices with a single minute of MOVE. By breaking down healthy behaviors into moment-by-moment, minute-by-minute decisions and actions, you can always make a choice to do what's good for your overall well-being. Health journeys are never linear paths. They are winding, and messy. Just keep moving forward!

3.5 Choose to be embodied

The ThinkMOVE program helps you reintegrate the mind and the body so they are one whole. It moves away from the pattern of being a body at the gym and a brain staring at a computer all day at work. Body awareness is the practice of listening to how you feel (tensions, emotions, stress) and noticing how you are using your body (e.g., posture, sitting for extended periods, hunger). Being embodied means being connected to yourself and your health in all environments.

The choice to be embodied looks like practicing healthy choices every day multiple times a day, whether that means taking the stairs, eating fruit, or disrupting prolonged sitting. It also means letting go of old patterns of relating to the body as an object to be molded and mended to meet society's expectations. There's a reason those exercise programs and fad diets never worked. Rather than thinking about what your body needs to look like to meet other people's expectations, being embodied means listening to what the body needs at the root of its being and doing that. The focus with being embodied is health. Reaching a healthy weight is a natural consequence of this practice.

3.6 Choose to connect

I encourage you to form teams of three to five people. Mastering movement at work is helped by having a positive and supportive social context. By focusing on social connection, you can face the barriers to movement at the workplace together. The community you create can be a powerful way of giving and receiving support. Fun team challenges and friendly competitions can help increase motivation.

Within your community at work, it is important that people are safe, which means no judgments or teasing comments. One of the biggest concerns I hear from people about to start the program is their worry that others will judge them. Each team member should try his or her best and offer support and encouragement to others.

3.7 Choose to MOVE in ways that work for you

Everything in ThinkMOVE is customizable because everyone is different. It's important to be sensitive to individual differences and limitations surrounding movement. Every element of the program can be adjusted, whether it's MOVEs per day, modifying specific exercises, or finding unique triggers. It is important that you find a way to create your own program that fits your body and lifestyle.

If there's an exercise in the program you don't like or you don't feel you can do safely, don't do it. Choose the exercises that you feel comfortable with and that you enjoy doing at your workplace. Listen to your body and respect your limits. Movement is an enjoyable experience. Our bodies can do so much. Taking a minute to move and appreciate the body can be energizing and healing itself.

3.8 Choose compelling goals

Keep in mind your important reasons for prioritizing your health and wanting to move more. Having clear goals that are compelling and meaningful to you and your team can help elevate motivation. The Exercise 17 in Chapter 9 will help you set realistic and achievable goals.

Why is health important for you? What are you hoping to experience through the ThinkMOVE program? How will those you love be impacted if you were healthier?

3.9 Choose to be positive

One of our missions is to take the guilt out of health and exercise and replace it with experiences of fun, mastery, and connection. Taking care of our health doesn't have to be a painful chore. So often we think about health negatively: the weight we want to lose, the foods we need to stop eating, the exercise we're not getting. With ThinkMOVE, you can create a positive vision of your health. Off-days can be moments of learning, and growth can be measured mostly by people's willingness to return to the practice of movement.

Along any healthy journey, you are bound to experience negativity. Keeping a positive mindset which includes acceptance, compassion, and growth is necessary to overcome setbacks and challenges.

3.10 Choose to have fun

Learn to laugh at yourself and not take things so seriously. The Think-MOVE program has challenges for individuals and teams to keep them engaged and motivated. It will help you work more efficiently, leaving you with more time and energy to do important things outside of work like connecting with friends and family.

4. MOVE-ing at Work Isn't a Break from Work: It Is a WAY of Working

ThinkMOVE is a new way of working, one that helps address health and the needs of the body while also improving work performance by using movement to create a sustainable work rhythm that optimizes energy.

Movement can be used to improve the quality of our work. We can have standing meetings where we are free to move or stretch anytime. We can go for walking meetings where we can gain the benefits of movement and being outside to stimulate our brains and enhance the quality and efficiency of meetings.

Many times throughout this book we have made reference to MOVE breaks. To be clear, taking a MOVE break doesn't always mean taking a break from work, it means primarily taking a break from sitting. We encourage you to use the MOVE break as a way of moving deeper into your work and moving past stuck points. For example, if you're struggling with formulating an email, you could try doing some squats. Doing some exercise can help open up perspectives, get the blood flowing, and inspire new ideas.

We are not machines and can't expect to be on all the time. MOVE breaks are also mental breaks that enable us to recover from periods of work. In strength training, rest is an important aspect of any workout. It enables a person to train at maximum output. We can think of taking a break from work periodically as a means of maintaining maximum focus and effort. If a person tries to work without taking a break, performance inevitably deteriorates along with health.

ThinkMOVE can become the secret ingredient that helps boost performance in all areas of your life. Here are some specific examples. ThinkMOVE is:

- a way into work (initiating work; starting is sometimes the hardest part)

- a fresh perspective on work (shifting: Thinking can get stagnant. Physical movement can help you break out of stuck points)

- a connector to colleagues, fostering a sense of belonging, when practiced as a team

- a way of improving focus at work (attention and emotion regulation)

- the goodness of a workout spread over the course of a day (improved health and fitness)

- a mood booster (increasing the production of mood boosting neurotransmitters: serotonin, dopamine, and norepinephrine)

- a stress buster (helps you get through stuck points)

- an energy manager (regular rest periods enable you to maintain a high level of focus and productivity)

The aphorism "a rising tide lifts all boats" fits well with the Think-MOVE program. We believe the success of ThinkMOVE will depend heavily on a company's ability to build a nurturing and supportive community amongst all members in the program. Just like with Weight Watchers®, whenever an individual is making a significant change in their lifestyle the support group model has proven to be a very important environmental factor in helping people change. The structure and accountability of the ThinkMOVE program is designed t̶ ͟ ͟re that you are not only learning the concepts, but bringing the ͟ ͟ ͟on at your workplace.

Exercise 5
Where Are You?

At what stage of change do you think you are?

Which of the ten resistances to movement apply to you?

Which of the ten choices to help you move might help you address re̶ plans or actions can you take to overcome resistance?

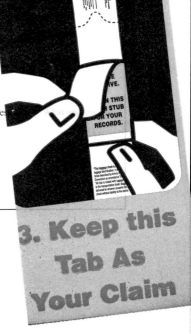

6

An Overview of the ThinkMOVE Program

So far, I've talked about how MOVE was created, reviewed research that shows the negative impact of sitting, analyzed the cultural context which makes sitting so prominent and being healthy so difficult, and reviewed the research behind ThinkMOVE.

Now I'd like to orient you to the different components of the program so you'll know what to expect and how to make the most of it for yourself or your team.

> **The ThinkMOVE program and Weight Loss**
>
> As discussed earlier, the body naturally compensates for large bouts of exercise by consuming increased calories. Many people can relate to the experience of finishing a tough workout and then feeling really hungry and entitled to indulge in something that's not healthy. This pattern offsets any of the benefits of working out in the first place! If losing weight is an important goal for you, ThinkMOVE is an effective adjunct to a healthy diet and exercise plan. Many early adopters have experienced weight loss through the program although that wasn't their primary goal.

Short bouts of exercises as in the ThinkMOVE program have been designed to increase caloric expenditure and metabolism without also increasing appetite. Other studies have been shown that short bouts of exercise before meals increase GLUT4 receptors which help transport more glucose into the muscle cells for energy instead of storing it as fat. We highly recommend participants practice doing either strength- or cardio-based MOVEs before meals to stimulate GLUT4 receptors and rev up their metabolism.

Not only will MOVE help increase your metabolism, it can also increase self-awareness regarding food choices. Many participants who have practiced MOVE before meals shared that just thinking about doing something healthy right before eating helped them make better choices.

Using an investment metaphor, we can think of these small increments of MOVE breaks as small financial investments. Over time, these small contributions add up by spreading the positive benefits of exercise and healthy choices over the course of your entire day. Before the MOVE program, a typical office worker could go through an entire day without a single constructive thought or action towards health.

1. What Is a MOVE Break?

A MOVE break is any disruption of sedentary time with movement which benefits your physical and mental health.

2. The Goals of the ThinkMOVE Program

The goal of the program is for participants to experience health and vitality in the workplace and throughout all areas of their lives.

Our primary goal is to work well and be well. MOVE does this by helping you become aware of what your body needs and giving you the tools and skills to take care of those needs. The foundational step is creating a connection between your mind and body: Think + MOVE!

Health improvements can be organized into three major categories:

1. **Physical health:** By making health the foundation for everything we do, we can be more effective and efficient. Our bodies will feel more loose, vital, and free.

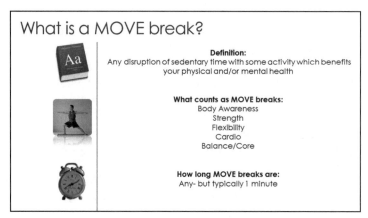

Figure 15

2. **Mental health:** By reconnecting body and mind, the work of the mind is supported by increased blood flow, increased metabolism, and increased flow of mood-boosting neurotransmitters. By freeing the body, you free the mind with noticeable improvements in focus, energy, mood, and productivity.

3. **Organizational health:** The program creates a structure where everyone is supporting each other towards optimizing their health. Health then becomes the foundation for accomplishing the company's mission and vision. People will feel more connected through a sense of shared purpose and belonging at the workplace regardless of different roles and departments.

3. Who is ThinkMOVE for?

ThinkMOVE can benefit almost anyone living and working a typical Western sedentary fashion. That being said, here is a list of characteristics that best describes the ideal ThinkMOVE participant:

- Works in an office and spends a majority of time sitting.

- Has experienced the negative effects of being sedentary: weight gain, low mood, low energy, and loss of focus/productivity.

- Has tried many different fitness regimes and has some knowledge of what works and doesn't work for him or her.

- Is less focused on body image and more concerned with health.

- Has noticed the effects of aging on the body and wants to learn to live with vitality well into his or her golden years!

To MOVE, you definitely don't need to be a huge health nut! Of course it would help if you were motivated to improve your overall health, but the practices of ThinkMOVE are accessible to a majority of people because they are very simple and convenient to do.

4. The Five Elements of MOVE

The ThinkMOVE program has been designed to address five core elements of physical and mental health, which look at the individual as a whole rather than focusing on one element such as "looking good." These are:

1. Body awareness
2. Strength
3. Cardio
4. Flexibility
5. Balance/core

Week by week, the program introduces basic MOVEs for each of these categories and later ensures that each week contains a balance of each of the five core elements. Here's why each of these elements are important and their real-world application is, in the following sections.

4.1 Body awareness

Many participants of ThinkMOVE report an inability to sit for long periods of time once they have been involved in the program. They share their newfound awareness of back stiffness or pain when sitting for a long time. How can this be? The ThinkMOVE program helps you become more aware of the effects of sitting and the needs of your body. It's not new pain but pain that's gone below the surface of awareness because you stopped paying attention. By moving, you create a contrasting experience and become more sensitive to the effects of prolonged sitting. Body awareness MOVEs can incorporate mindfulness meditation, visualization, guided relaxation, and coaching.

4.2 Strength

The average adult male loses one pound of muscle every year after the age of 30. Strength training helps preserve muscle. Strength training is also important for bone health, and functional strength for situations like lifting groceries, pushing heavy doors, and picking up your kids or grandkids. Strength MOVEs are based on traditional strength training, resistance bands, free-hand exercises, and kettlebell exercises.

4.3 Cardio

Being sedentary slows down every vital function: cardiovascular, digestive, and musculoskeletal. Doing cardio MOVEs ignites and stimulates these systems and reduces the risk of heart disease, diabetes, and cancer. Finally, in doing cardio MOVEs, we increase our energy which improves our ability to keep up with kids, to take the stairs, to chase after streetcars, and participate in other daily events without issue. Cardio MOVEs are a combination of traditional cardio, sports, boxing, capoeira, aerobic movements, and dance.

4.4 Flexibility

As you sit, you stiffen. Flexibility MOVEs help keep you limber; they also help prevent injury and improve or maintain your full range of motion. Plus stretching feels good and when you feel good you do good! Flexibility MOVEs draw from static and dynamic types of stretches as well as yoga.

4.5 Balance/core

We use balance all the time. Balance is essentially your ability to negotiate your body between your feet using your entire body. If you weren't able to balance and coordinate your body, you would just sag to the floor like a wet noodle. Balance is important for many daily functions like walking, going up stairs, getting in and out of the car, hopping over puddles, putting on socks/pants, and walking. Working on balance is key to preventing injury and maintaining mobility into your golden years. Core/Balance MOVEs are a combination of traditional core exercises like planking, yoga, martial arts, and sports.

5. Psychological Benefits of the Five Core Elements

Each of the five elements corresponds to particular psychological benefits in addition to physical benefits. As you begin to incorporate movement into your day, be intentional about what you want to get out of your MOVE break. Determine for yourself what psychological and/or physical benefits you hope to experience.

5.1 Body awareness

Body awareness exercises form the foundation for the other categories by creating the connection between mind and body. By practicing body awareness, the ability to listen to your body improves and you can better identify what it needs whether that is a MOVE break, rest, food, or social connection. So often we are pulled in a thousand directions throughout our day. Slowing down and listening to your whole body helps create an internal sense of centredness and groundedness. Taking a moment to breathe or tune into your body helps increase self awareness as well as your ability to focus, since you learn to self-direct your attention rather than always being other-directed.

All MOVE breaks are about self-care, and body awareness MOVEs are foundational to that. When you do a body awareness MOVE (whether that's listening to your body, increasing the length of your breath, or improving posture), remind yourself that these are acts of self-love and self-nurturance that help strengthen you.

Intention: Self-care.

5.2 Strength

Strength MOVEs are similar in nature to core/balance exercises. They incorporate more dynamic movement and the pushing, pulling, lifting of resistance. We encourage participants to challenge themselves to move their bodies through the fullest range of motion they are capable of. Strength training increases lean muscle and muscle tonality resulting in increased confidence. With improved strength, you are more able to hold your body in a healthy position (i.e., abs and glutes engaged, and shoulders back) rather than slouching. When you hold yourself with more confidence, you inevitably feel more confident and appear that way to others. As the saying goes, "When you look good, you feel good, and when you feel good, you do good!" With every strength MOVE, you are practicing overcoming resistance and thereby feeling stronger and improving willpower.

Intention: Persistence, strength (literally).

5.3 Cardio

The very act of pausing your work is challenging enough. There is a temptation in the workplace to carry on mindlessly without paying attention to what you are doing, how you are doing, and what is a priority. Cardio MOVEs increase blood flow to our brains (including the prefrontal cortex, which improves focus and problem solving). Some participants in the ThinkMOVE program use cardio MOVEs as a way to break out of stuck points in their work and generate energy when they are feeling tired. Cardio MOVEs can be a tool for increasing persistence, endurance, and mental energy. Sometimes when we get stuck in our work we might procrastinate. By pausing and doing a MOVE, you are training yourself to continue even when it is difficult. The physical movement gives your mind a mental break to gain some perspective and return to the work with fresh eyes and energizing endorphins!

Intention: Persistence; generating energy.

5.4 Flexibility

With every MOVE we teach, we also encourage mental awareness. Flexibility MOVEs are a natural place to practice this, as you may have experienced if you've ever done a yoga class. Flexibility MOVEs are done slowly and intentionally. Focusing on deep breathing will help release unnecessary tension. Practicing flexibility can help cultivate calmness, relaxation, a flexible mindset, and going with the flow.

Intention: Stretching limits, going with the flow.

5.5 Balance

Most balance MOVEs are static. They involve holding a particular pose such as a plank or standing on one foot for as long as possible. These exercises strengthen your core stabilizer muscles that are not used at all when you are engulfed in a chair or couch. Core/balance MOVEs help increase focus and concentration as well as ability to regulate emotions, since it is frustrating when you lose your balance. Practice persistence through the coordination of all parts of your body and find that place of balance that enables you to hold the position with poise and ease.

Intention: Focus and balancing effort with effortlessness.

Chair Pose

Challenge yourself to do a chair pose where you pretend to be sitting on an invisible chair for as long as possible. Chair pose is a strength move and is a great opportunity to build mental strength in the face of challenge. Hold the pose and allow yourself to go through the various challenging stages. In the beginning,

---

you may feel slight discomfort but gradually, you will feel the lactic acid build up into a burning sensation in your legs. You will be tempted to stop. Don't give into this temptation right away! Try to keep going as long as possible.

This is an example of a strength MOVE that pushes you to overcome the mental impulse to quit. Any physical challenge we experience is inevitably a psychological challenge as well. Learn to listen to your thoughts and feelings and coach yourself to keep calm and persist. You will sharpen the body and mind.

6. Sustainable Engagement with MOVE, or Creating a Long-Term Relationship with Your Health

Many exercise programs are framed within 30 to 90 days with no concrete plan beyond that time period. Developing the MOVE-ing habit takes time. In my practice, we like to work with our clients for at least six months to ensure they have a good grasp of the MOVE system and the culture shift to take place.

People need a vision for how they can maintain their health gains in the long term. The initial ThinkMOVE program lays the foundation for health and movement at the office. Once participants have learned the basic skills, they move on to more advanced programming which enables them to stay moving for years! Health is a lifelong journey. With each stage of life we need to adapt and learn new ways of challenging our bodies and maintaining good health.

As participants progress beyond the introductory stages they learn how to integrate the five dimensions of body awareness, flexibility, strength, core/balance, and cardio. For example, in round two of Flexibility, flexibility MOVEs will be combined with strength in one MOVE break. This might mean doing lunges while in warrior pose. By integrating the five elements together, participants challenge the body in new ways and integrate them without increasing the time needed to practice.

As companies progress, we teach participants how to create their own workouts lasting anywhere between 5 to 60 minutes using the exercises they have learned. Acute bouts of exercise have their place in improving athletic performance as well as maintaining weight loss.

We want to encourage participants to love health and fitness and we see the MOVE program as an excellent jumping-off point for people to become accustomed and familiar with exercise in bite-sized pieces.

7. Program Orientation

Materials you will need:

1. ThinkMOVE book/journal or ThinkMOVE application to record activities. (See the download kit for a journal you can use or www.thinkmove.ca for the app.)

2. Triggering tools (phone alarm, paper, or electronic agenda).

3. Enough space by your desk or in your office to MOVE!

4. A resistance band (optional).

The MOVE system is essentially three steps:

1. Trigger the break using a reminder such as a scheduled alert or a situational trigger.

2. Input what exercise/MOVE you will be doing in your Think-MOVE journal or the MOVE application.

3. MOVE! Take that minute to do your MOVE exercise and return to work more energized and focused.

In addition to body awareness and the other four categories of MOVE (flexibility, strength, balance, and cardio) participants learn specific skills which enable them to disrupt sedentary time. These include:

7.1 Triggering skills

This is a basic overview of triggering skills.

- **Scheduling trigger** (week one): Set aside specific times in your day to do MOVE breaks. Use your alarm or agenda to trigger. This is the most basic triggering tool.

- **Feelings and physical sensations triggers** (week two): Use common recurring events to trigger the act of moving, e.g., when the phone rings, stand up and do squats.

- **Stringing** (week four): Stringing is the most important tool used in the MOVE program to consistently disrupt long periods of sedentary time. It is also a productivity tool that helps you manage your energy and stay focused on your work. More on this later.

7.2 Celebrating/appreciating your efforts

The ability to celebrate yourself, your efforts, and your accomplishments is a skill. Celebrating or appreciating yourself might seem odd especially in our culture but doing so strengthens you and makes it more likely that you will continue to practice. The media typically depicts exercise as a harsh and militant experience like on the show *The Biggest Loser* where trainers scream and berate contestants. With ThinkMOVE, we take a completely different approach, one that emphasizes positivity, nurturance, and effort. Celebrating sustains the effort.

Don't fall into the self-critic trap. Every time you finish a MOVE break, give yourself credit! You're doing something good for your health both physically and mentally; you deserve some credit and thanks.

There are a few simple ways that you can incorporate celebration into your MOVE habit.

1. Celebrate each MOVE. Every time you complete a MOVE break, acknowledge your efforts by saying: "That was great!" or a simple "thank you" to yourself for taking the time to care for your body. Another way might be to connect to the positive feelings or physiological sensations of doing the MOVE break (e.g., "I feel more energized now!," "I feel more calm/relaxed/less stressed," "I feel stronger now that I've used my muscles."

2. Celebrate with your friends. Do a MOVE break with a friend and give each other some positive feedback. "Nice squat!," "Good job!," a high-five, "You're rad!" It may seem cheesy because we rarely celebrate ourselves and each other publicly. We work hard every day, and jump from one task to the next leaving little time to celebrate our efforts and accomplishments. Try it, I promise it won't hurt, it will feel great!

3. Celebrate the total number of MOVES you achieve by the end of the day or week. Even if you don't meet your goal, realize that every minute you do is a minute you would have been sitting. Something is always better than nothing especially when research is showing that simple disruptions of sitting can address the sedentary problem.

4. Celebrate the changes you make. You may notice in the first week or two that your awareness of your body changes and you feel more connected. You may notice that your breathing is getting deeper and your posture healthier. Notice the milestones that you achieve and celebrate these.

How many MOVES Per Day (MPD) should I aim to do?

Tracking the number of MOVEs you do each day is the most important and relevant information for the purpose of this program. Research has demonstrated that the issue with sitting is not sitting per se but prolonged periods of uninterrupted sitting. Since that is the case, breaks or disruptions of sitting that amount to short bouts of exercise or healthy movement are excellent ways to break up that sitting time and stimulate the various systems across the body including digestive, cardiovascular, hormonal, and musculoskeletal to name a few.

There are two major ways of tracking MPD: either through the MOVE application which provides users with timers and an archive of exercises, or a MOVE journal which people can keep with them throughout their days. See the download kit for a journal you can use.

You might be wondering, "How many MOVE breaks do I need to do every day?" It depends on how much sitting you do per day. As a general rule, research is suggesting that you should be taking a break from sitting every 20–30 minutes.

You can do a few quick calculations to set your minimum, ideal, maximum number (first determine how many hours a day you sit per day):

- If you sit 10 hours a day your minimum would be 1x10 hours = 10 MPD (i.e., a break every hour)

- If you sit 10 hours a day your ideal would be 2x10 = 20 MPD (i.e., a break every 30 minutes)

- If you sit 10 hours a day it would be 3x10 = 30 MPD (i.e., a break every 20 minutes)

These numbers represent where people could be when they have achieved a certain level of mastery with the MOVE system. The program begins at a modest 3 MPD and increases by one MOVE each week. At the end of the six weeks, participants are challenged to average around 7 MPD, which is very good and leaves lots of room to grow. Participants with an average of 6.5 MPD improved their strength, cardio, and flexibility as well as their energy, focus and productivity at the end of just nine weeks. Any disruption of sitting time is going to have positive impact as it disrupts the total number of hours of sitting per day.

It takes time to build the moving habit (anywhere from six months to a year). We have had years, decades even, of training in schools, later at work, to sit still and not fidget or move. The MOVE program challenges the sitting habit by encouraging the practice of listening and tuning into the body's needs and respecting them as they arise instead of ignoring them.

8. Program Weekly Outline

Each weekly section that follows is organized into three parts: lesson, exercises, and practice.

8.1 Lesson

Each week focuses on a specific health topic. As mentioned, our first core element is body awareness, which is creating the connection between body and mind. Other topics will include healthy breathing and healthy positions.

8.2 Exercises

This section will include all of the new MOVE exercises for the week. We begin with body awareness and then flexibility, balance, strength, and cardio in subsequent weeks, then we put them together.

8.3 Practice

You will be given specific triggers, exercises, and MOVEs per day challenges every week. All of these practices happen in one or two minute breaks throughout your day.

9. Keep Calm and Move On

When you try something new, there can be pressure to perform. As you introduce movement into your day, keep the intention of being calm and relaxed. Don't create tension or stress. This is not meant to be another pressure-filled task for the to-do list. It's a chance to inject your day with energizing breaks which enhance your work. An opportunity to nurture the body and the mind so you can be healthy.

INTERNAL TRIGGERS	EXTERNAL TRIGGERS
• FEELINGS	• TIME (SCHEDULING)
• PHYSICAL SENSATIONS	• ENVIRONMENTAL
• THOUGHTS	• SOCIAL
• BEHAVIOR	• TOOLS (APPS)

Figure 16

Before doing a MOVE break, try to take a few deep, relaxing breaths so that you are putting your mind and body in a positive state and moving away from stress.

10. Week One: Body Awareness

In week one we focus on body awareness.

Objectives this week:

- To begin to listen to the body and hear what it needs.

- To learn the process of body awareness and the different windows from which to become aware.

- To practice getting up from a seated position and paying attention to the body.

- To learn about the eight different types of triggers that can prompt movement.

- To use scheduling triggers three to four times per day as a way to begin MOVE breaks.

- For the team to practice moving together and feeling connected and supported with each other.

We'll also be learning and practicing MOVEs from the other elements of strength, flexibility, core/balance, and cardio. However, becoming aware of our bodies is the first step to developing the moving habit.

Body awareness is the conscious practice of creating and maintaining a connection between your mind and the rest of your body.

Body awareness practices help us undo the splitting of mind and body that happens when we work sitting down all day. Our current sedentary lifestyles have created this artificial divide between the mind and body because in the office we focus on mental work without much physical activity. We reserve movement and consideration of the body for the gym if we consider it at all. As previously discussed, we can see how we have evolved from being a movement-based organism to one where the separation of movement from our environment has created an artificial separation of mind and body.

Specifically, body awareness is the skill of paying attention to the sensations of the body so that you can identify what you are feeling (emotions), how you are using your body (position), and choices about what to do to be healthier (specific exercises).

Imagine driving a car that has no dashboard, no speedometer, tachometer, gas, oil light, signaling light/sound, or temperature gauge of the engine. How would you feel about driving this car? All the displays that we take for granted are important parts of the driving experience. Each display contains information that we use to drive well and safely.

The human body may not come with a visual dashboard, but we are constantly receiving signals from our bodies. Body awareness is learning to tune in and listen to these signals.

The ThinkMOVE program helps you reintegrate all the parts of your body as a congruent whole by incorporating regular movement breaks throughout the day. By learning how to listen to your body and creating an internal connection to it, you'll be able to identify what it needs, whether that be rest or specific moves, moment by moment. Body awareness is a foundational skill that will empower you to reach your health goals.

Exercise 6
Body Awareness

Let's try a short body awareness exercise.

Take a moment to ask yourself: "How is my body feeling right now?" Notice the position of your body and any sensations of soreness/stiffness. Notice where your body makes contact with the chair and how comfortable or uncomfortable this position is. Notice any sensations happening inside. Are you feeling tired, hungry, energized?

By becoming aware of your body and its current state you can become more skilled in offering what it needs, whether that be movement, rest, or food. Also, the very act of paying attention and listening to the body helps nurture and strengthen it.

Cultivating body awareness helps individuals understand the connection between their subjective experience of thoughts, feelings, and stress and their physiology. By increasing awareness of the body's signal of tiredness, worry, stress, soreness, stiffness, and responding skillfully, participants tend to experience major benefits. You can:

- Become fully embodied (create space for your body at work).

- Reduce soreness and stiffness in your body.

- Increase self-awareness.

- Identify your needs and take care of them (e.g., I'm tired I need to do some cardio to boost my energy).

- Create natural internal triggers (e.g., feeling stuck means I need to take a minute to move and come back to this problem).

- Become more self-directed (you are the boss and expert of you and your body).

- Learn to value and appreciate your body. Rather than focusing on what's wrong or what you want to change, you'll practice nurturing yourself so you can grow yourself.

- Increase your capacity to cope with work demands and stress.

- Increase your ability to relax and go with the flow.

- Gain confidence in your self-care abilities.

- Other _____

10.1 Week one lesson: Steps to body awareness

1. Breathing

2. Attending

3. Relaxing

4. Letting go of tension

5. Appreciating

These five steps are a general outline of how to become aware of your body. This is only a guideline to begin developing body awareness. Relaxing and letting go are the steps to processing those experiences and appreciating is a way of anchoring the practice and ending.

With practice, you will find that you don't need to follow this specific order. Instead you can do the elements that feel right for you in a sequence that fits for your body. In other words, you can interact and engage your body creatively.

As much as possible, try to do the body awareness exercises from a standing position.

Exercise 7
Benefits and Steps to Body Awareness

Benefits of Body Awareness

• **Improved mind and body connection:**
  • By increasing awareness, participants will create a healthy relationship with their bodies and minds; one that includes appreciation and respect for all that it does and makes possible.
  • Individuals will feel more connected, more whole, more vital and as a result they will be able to think better, listen better, communicate better, and work better.

• **Improved mental health:**
  • Increased energy, willpower, and focus.
  • Improved ability to be in the present moment.
  • Increased capacity to deal with demands and stress.
  • Increase in positive mood.
  • Increased capacity and skills to cope with stress and demands.
  • The ability to take breaks and gain perspective and shift out of stuck points.

• **Reduction of body soreness, tension, and stiffness:**
  • Participants will learn skills to perform healthy and needed body maintenance so aches and pains are addressed and they experience comfort and mobility. Remember, "motion is lotion."
  • Increased ability to relax the body and go with the flow.
  • Improved posture and movement patterns.

Personalized Goals for Body Awareness
Goals for improving body awareness can include:
(Place a checkmark beside the goals that are important to you.)

	Improved breath awareness and deeper breathing
	Increased self-awareness
	Increased mindfulness; ability to be present and focused
	Improved mood; less anxiety or depression
	Increased energy and productivity
	A healthier relationship with the body
	Reducing soreness/stiffness in the body
	Increased moments of calmness and relaxation
	Improved posture while sitting, standing, walking, and exercising
	Reduced tension throughout the body; increased relaxation
	Others:

We begin with the breath. Notice how you are breathing (deep or shallow) and then take some deep calming breaths to ground yourself. Our breath is the anchor that brings us back into our bodies.

Simply notice how you are breathing for a few breaths without trying to change it. When you are ready, begin to take deep gentle breaths. Do this four or five times. Aim for a ratio of three seconds for the inhalation and four seconds for exhalation. Research shows that a slower exhalation can help calm the nervous system and lower your heart rate, which is important when coping with stress.

Next, we focus on attending to the rest of the body and this is done primarily by asking yourself, "What am I feeling in my body right now?"

There are six main windows from which to listen into the body:

1. Feelings/physical sensations

2. Breathing

3. Attention

4. Tensions

5. Posture/body position

6. Movement

See Exercise 8.

Exercise 8
Questions to Ask Yourself That Will Give You Windows into Body Awareness

Feelings/physical sensations	What am I feeling right now? What's going on in my stomach and heart areas? How do my legs feel?
Breathing	How am I breathing right now? Shallow/deep, fast/slow, nose/mouth?
Attention	Where is my focus and attention right now?
Tension	Where is there tension in my body right now?
Posture/body position	How am I holding my body right now? What position am I in? Am I comfortable or uncomfortable? Do I need to move?
Movement	You will learn various movements in this program including flexibility, balance, strength, and cardio. Each movement is a way of listening and understanding the body. You might ask: "How does it feel to do a flexibility move right now? What is happening in my body and what changes do I notice both physically and mentally?"

You'll notice that breathing is listed both as part of the process of becoming body aware and as a window into body awareness. It is both a tool to help you listen to feelings and physical sensations as well as an important process to pay attention to on its own. Try to be intentional about the way you are using breath, either as a vehicle to observe your body (e.g., lengthening the breath and expanding the lungs in order to notice tensions in the body) or as something to watch itself (i.e., the depth of your breathing, the pace).

As you become aware of the windows into the body, you can practice relaxing the body and letting go of any excessive tensions you notice along the way. Connected to breathing is the ability to relax. The breath is one simple and powerful way to bring relaxation to the body. Whenever you exhale during the practice, imagine softening all your muscles including your neck, shoulders, arms, and face. Let your skeletal structure hold you up instead of your muscles and use the minimum amount of muscle tone to stay upright. As you do this you might notice particular areas of tension. Use your breath to expand these areas and imagine letting go of the tension on the next exhalation.

As you attend to your body, notice your body position/posture. Poor posture can often create a lot of tension in the body. Becoming aware of where muscles are overused or in bad positions can lead to better decisions and a lessening of tension. Relaxation is a central theme that runs through all body awareness exercises.

When you are finished, take a moment to appreciate what you have done for your body before ending the practice. You have connected to your breath, attended to your body, relaxed, and let go of tension. The final step is the practice of appreciating and celebrating the body. This might mean recognizing and appreciating what's healthy and good about the body including the signals of pain, soreness, or stiffness that are calling for your attention. This could be as simple as reflecting on a few specific things that are going well with your body or it could be noting the change you feel after practicing body awareness.

10.2 Week one exercise: Body awareness

The body awareness process is a part of all MOVE exercises whether it be flexibility, strength, cardio, or balance. When doing any MOVE, it is important to be aware of what is happening both physically and psychologically to get the most from the exercise. For example, while doing a strength movement, it is important to be tuned into one's breathing in order to let go of unneeded tension and to be aware of which muscles are being used and how they are moving.

It is challenging to be open to all the body awareness windows while moving. That's why in week one we simply practice this while standing. Although you could attend to a mix of breath, physical sensations, attention, tensions, and posture, I would suggest this week focusing on feelings and physical sensations. If you are someone who sits for long periods, noticing your feelings and physical sensations will be challenging and likely give you plenty of motivation to disrupt sitting time. Have fun playing with these tools and skills. Take your time with each window as you notice what each one has to communicate.

Listening might make you aware of old pain

Practicing listening to your body and reconnecting to it throughout the day may mean that you become aware of painful sensations that went unnoticed. Often people tell me they can't sit for long periods anymore because they become so aware of how painful it is to lock the body up in the seated position. Feeling your pain signals is like being able to see the traffic signals while you drive. They are necessary messages about how to take care of your body. Without them we end up crashing into telephone poles or burnt out from driving the body beyond its limits.

This week you won't be learning any specific movements. The most critical element is learning to listen and to get up from your seat.

You are going to start listening authentically to your body, then applying various types of movements that fit for you and what your body needs in the present moment. This practice positions you as the expert of your body. That makes sense because you experience you from the inside out. Everyone else is an outsider, including so-called experts.

For this week simply standing up and listening to your body is enough of a practice. It doesn't sound like much, but standing up (or taking a stand against sitting!) creates a contrasting experience that allows you to feel the shifts in the body. When you go through the various windows into the body you'll notice how just standing up can change the way you feel, the way you breathe, and how present you are.

This week is about taking stock of your body and evaluating the impact of sitting on your health. There's no need to rush into any movement exercises since you have the rest of your life to practice. The important step is to develop awareness of your body and everything that is taking place within it right now. Don't rush or skip this step of becoming body aware.

In addition to each body awareness exercise you do, feel free to do whatever movement or stretch you are already comfortable and familiar with and input these into the ThinkMOVE app to track.

10.3 Week one practice

You will learn a series of triggers that will help you initiate move breaks seamlessly throughout your day. Internal triggers relate to your subjective experience as it occurs within your body. External triggers have to do with the environment and involve tools or support from others.

We will go into more depth each week regarding each trigger type. For now, there is a quick summary of each trigger in Figure 17.

Trigger Type	Example
*Feelings (Internal Trigger)	Feeling stressed, unfocused, or overwhelmed
*Psychological sensations (Internal Trigger)	Feeling sore, tired, thirsty, stiff
*Thoughts	"I can't get this all done today!"
*Behavior (Internal Trigger)	Yawning, phone calls, posture is slouched
Time (External Trigger)	Lunch time, 3:00 p.m. (This trigger is covered with scheduling of week 1.)
Environmental (External Trigger)	At water cooler, meeting, microwaving, after a long drive
Social interactions (External Trigger)	Coworker comes to visit you or you want to connect
Tools (apps)	Pomodoro Timers, ThinkMOVE app

Feelings, psychological sensations, thoughts, and behavior are triggers that relate to and enhance body awareness. Paying attention to these is an important part of connecting the mind and body.

Figure 17

These trigger categories are the basic elements of any situation. Although they are occurring simultaneously all the time, we can prioritize certain elements as a reminder to do a MOVE break. Feelings, physical sensations, and behavior are internal triggers meaning they are based on our subjective experience or actions. Environments and social interactions are external triggers meaning they involve some kind of outside interaction. They occur outside of us and are not within our control but they can be used to help trigger MOVE breaks.

For example, you may be feeling tired (physical) and unfocused (feeling). You notice the time is 3:00 p.m. (time) and you realize that you usually feel tired at this time. You are at work (environment) and you have been sitting alone (social) for hours (behavior). In this example, the feeling of being tired might be the primary trigger that you use to become aware of needing to take a MOVE break.

Any of the trigger types can be the primary trigger. As you practice, it is helpful to become aware of the other elements that occur in connection to your primary trigger since it makes the trigger more memorable and powerful.

There are many opportunities to integrate MOVEs into your day. There is a list of possibilities in Exercise 9.

Exercise 9
Triggers

Take a moment to check off all the situational triggers you might use to prompt a MOVE break.

ANYTIME:

- [ ] after going to the bathroom while washing hands (hold chair pose)
- [ ] sitting in office meetings (stealth MOVES)
- [ ] taking the stairs (functional lunges)
- [ ] getting in and out of car (practice engaging your core)
- [ ] talking to someone in person (go for walking meeting or do a quick stretch!)
- [ ] talking to someone on the phone (squats)
- [ ] in a bathroom stall while at a restaurant (squats to rev up metabolism)
- [ ] waiting in line (balance MOVE)
- [ ] feeling tired, sore, stiff, or pain in the body
- [ ] feeling stressed, stuck, or overwhelmed
- [ ] feeling unfocused or distracted
- [ ] your back feels sore
- [ ] showering (mindful moment)
- [ ] you notice your posture is slouched (practice a healthier position or MOVE)
- [ ] reaching for a cupboard (move mindfully and slowly)
- [ ] bending down to pick something up (practice a perfect squat or dead lift)
- [ ] while cooking, especially if you're just waiting for something to boil, sear, bake, etc. balance or cardio MOVE)
- [ ] checking your phone (just stand up for a minute!)
- [ ] checking Facebook, Twitter, email, etc. (stretch!)

MORNING

- [ ] waking up (dynamic stretches; morning wake-up routine)
- [ ] just before leaving for work do something more intense, cardio/strength MOVES to increase blood flow, oxygen, mental alertness, and clarity
- [ ] waiting for the kettle to boil/coffee to brew

- [ ] while waiting in line in a store (single leg squat)
- [ ] just after showering and before getting dressed (push ups)
- [ ] while brushing teeth (balancing on one foot)
- [ ] putting on clothes (squat while you button up your shirt)
- [ ] putting on underwear /socks /shoes/pants or any challenging pieces of clothes (balancing) just before breakfast (strength/cardio MOVE)
- [ ] working for extended periods at desk with a computer in office or cubicle (stringing technique taught in week 4)

AFTERNOON
- [ ] while microwaving lunch (jogging on the spot)
- [ ] having lunch (before each meal essentially) do 100 squats before each meal.
- [ ] during long staff meetings (stealth MOVES)
- [ ] whenever you are feeling tired or unfocused
- [ ] whenever you are feeling sore or stiff
- [ ] go for an afternoon walk with a coworker or on your own. Get outside, get some fresh air!
- [ ] do a cardio move to overcome the afternoon sleepy hour
- [ ] working for extended periods at desk with a computer in office or cubicle (stringing technique taught in week 4)

EVENING
- [ ] before or after dinner
- [ ] taking off clothes
- [ ] spending time with your kids (do something active like tag, dance, or wrestle)
- [ ] sitting on a couch watching TV (stretches; foam rolling)
- [ ] brushing teeth at night
- [ ] just before bed

10.4 MOVE skill: Scheduling

Scheduling is the first triggering technique taught in the MOVE program. It's easy to learn because everyone already knows how to schedule an appointment or a meeting. In the case of MOVE, you are simply scheduling mini-MOVE breaks with yourself or your team.

One of the challenges of scheduling MOVE breaks is you may not be in the habit of carving out time for your health. Also, it may not be the norm for your work culture yet, but hopefully the culture is shifting. Try to prioritize these meetings with yourself as you would an important staff or client meeting. It will only take a minute and it will help you create a healthier and more productive life. If it helps, perhaps schedule your MOVE breaks with someone on your team as a support.

The key to scheduling is that it should be at the START of the main sections of your day.

Here are some examples:

- First thing in the morning soon after waking (7:00 a.m.)
- When you start your day at work (9:00 a.m.)
- After lunch, when you start working again (1:00 p.m.)
- Midafternoon when you tend to feel tired (3:00 p.m.)
- At the start of the evening when you return home. (7:00 p.m.)

The reason I emphasize planting key times for MOVE is these become the main branches for accumulating MOVE breaks in combination with the other triggering techniques (situational and stringing). Starting can often times be the hardest part. Planting your three start times is integral to developing the moving habit.

Another way to use the scheduling trigger is to select times of the day when you know you are most stressed or sedentary.

Did you know?

A space shuttle uses more fuel in its first three minutes after liftoff than during its entire voyage around the earth?

In the same way, starting anything is often the hardest part. Start your day (or sections of your day, like early afternoon or early evening) with a MOVE break and know that just by starting you've won half the battle.

10.5 How to schedule MOVE breaks

1. Pick three regular times that would work for you to do one-minute MOVE breaks.

2. Choose and set up your scheduling method.

3. Practice doing your three MOVE breaks daily.

4. Appreciate yourself for practicing scheduling MOVE breaks daily. Before you return to your work, take a moment to celebrate the effort and attention you have given yourself. Notice the positive benefits pausing and getting connected to your body has had on your mind, mood, and body. You might note to yourself how you now feel: "I feel energized," or "I feel relaxed and focused." At the end of the week, you might give yourself a small reward to reinforce your efforts.

10.6 Scheduling methods

Here are a few ways to schedule MOVE breaks to increase the likelihood they will happen. Pick one or two to practice this week:

1. Schedule using the ThinkMOVE app.

2. Write it into your paper/digital agenda either daily or weekly (3x) and select times when you know you will have a minute.

3. Use a Post-It note and place it on by your desk or beside your computer screen.

4. Use a recurring alarm or email alert.

5. Connect with a colleague or your team and agree to meet for a MOVE break at regular times throughout the day. Commit to regular meetings.

6. You can also use a behavioral trigger to schedule a MOVE since there are routine behaviors you do on a daily basis. For example, while waiting for the computer to load up or for the coffee to brew. For some, it might be better and more natural to use some behavioral trigger to schedule a MOVE break. For others simply setting the time to start might work better. Experiment and decide which works best for you.

Try to do three to four MOVE BREAKS PER DAY (MPDs). Use the ThinkMOVE web application to input these breaks.

Use either the app or a daily journal such as what is shown in Exercise 10 to record your experience and reflections of the MOVE breaks. There is a journal on the download kit for you to use if you wish.

Exercise 10
Schedule

Write down your three scheduled MOVE times and scheduling method here:

Scheduled MOVE times	Scheduling Method
1.	
2.	
3.	

10.7 Move: Focus on body awareness

In the weeks to come, you'll be introduced to the other move categories of flexibility, balance, strength, and cardio.

This week you'll focus on practicing the four body awareness exercises you learned in this chapter for one to two minutes each time. Remember the steps for body awareness including connecting to your breath, listening to windows into the body, relaxing, letting go of tension, and appreciating your body.

Pay attention to the signals and sensations that appear in your body through each one. After each body awareness practice feel free to move, wiggle, and stretch in whatever way feels good and comfortable.

11. Week Two: Flexibility and Breathing

Our objectives for week two are to work on flexibility and breathing.

- Learn about the benefits of conscious and deeper breathing.
- Learn how to do belly breathing so that you can increase body awareness and create calm in your day.
- Learn a series of flexibility moves and reverse the effects of sitting.
- Use feeling/physical sensation triggers as a way of triggering MOVE breaks.
- Anticipate barriers to moving and support each other through these challenges.

11.1 Week two lesson

Healthy breathing is important. Our breath is our connection to life and a source of tremendous power. It is the pathway to becoming centered and grounded. Awareness and breath practice can help us regulate our physiology and emotions.

Our respiratory system is one of the few body functions we can consciously control or completely ignore. In either case, we would still live. It is a loyal friend. If you ever have the chance to observe an infant breathing you will see their little tummies expanding and contracting. Babies naturally breathe from their bellies, which is a deep, full breath. In yoga and most meditation practices this is called belly breathing; it is also called diaphragmatic breathing. Your diaphragm is a sheet of skeletal muscle that enables the lungs to draw air into the body.

Although belly breathing is the healthiest way to breathe, a great majority of us tend to breathe only into our chests or our necks by the time we reach adulthood. These short shallow breaths barely fill our lungs and provide only the bare minimum of oxygen to the rest of the body. Shallow breathing can lead to inadequate oxygen intake, which can make you feel lightheaded and weak. When a person experiences high levels of stress, their breathing can become even more shallow, when they remember to breathe at all! This creates stress on the body and reduces energy and vitality.

The quality of our breath is important to be aware of: Is my breathing rapid, shallow, or stuck? Is it calm, relaxed, and deep? What is the connection between how I am breathing and my thoughts, feelings, or situation? Also, the breath can be a tool for regulating emotion, improving willpower, and training attention.

Think of your breath as the front entrance to tuning into and becoming aware of all that is going on inside the house that is your body. Becoming aware of your breath enables you to become aware of your thoughts, feelings, physical tensions, and posture. Taking time to tune into your breath and practicing deep belly breathing helps create the space to listen to what is happening in the body. Often what is needed is deep breathing to stay calm, focused, and relaxed.

Research has shown that the practice of mindfully slowing down the breath can help increase willpower — the ability to control your attention, emotions, and desires. By creating calmness and groundedness through the breath, we can move away from reacting to situations and instead respond creatively and intelligently. The researchers found that long-term meditators had more gray matter in their prefrontal cortex, the area responsible for self-awareness and executive functions, including the ability to pay attention, regulate emotions, control impulses, problem solve, and learn.

This week you will learn practices that will help you bring calmness and relaxation into your life and connect it to the body. They will also help you improve regulation of emotions, self-control, and willpower.

11.1a Lengthening the breath: the practice of slowing and deepening breathing

One way that scientists have of measuring willpower is through heart rate variability (HRV). HRV is essentially small heart rate changes that happen between individual heartbeats, influenced by the way you breathe. Your heart speeds when you inhale and slows when you exhale. Higher variability is an indicator of health. Low variability is connected to things like heart failure, diabetic neuropathy, and mood disorders.

Research demonstrates that slowing your breathing rate helps increase HRV which is an important marker of health and improved willpower. For example, recovering alcoholics whose HRV goes up when they see a drink are more likely to stay sober. Recovering alcoholics who show the opposite response have a greater likelihood of relapsing. Other studies have also shown that people with higher HRV are better at ignoring distractions, delaying gratification, persisting in the face of failure, and dealing with stressful situations.

When we are under stress, the sympathetic nervous system takes over and we are into our fight or flight reactions. Our heart rate goes up and HRV goes down. When the heart gets "stuck" at low variability, it contributes to feeling angry, out of control, or overwhelmed as well as having a faster heart rate and increased blood pressure.

As mentioned, research shows that changing one's breathing rate can impact HRV. Specifically, the highest levels of heart rate variability occur in the range of four to six breaths per minute (BPM). Less than four BPM, heart rate variability decreases as it is likely causing stress on the body, not relaxation. Aim between four to six breaths per minute, but if you aren't yet able to get to four to six breaths per minute, don't worry. HRV increases as breathing drops below 12 breaths per minute.

Other factors that impact/influence HRV include anything that puts stress on the mind and body such as:

- Experiencing anger, anxiety, depression, or loneliness
- Chronic pain/illness
- Lack of exercise
- Poor sleep
- An unhealthy diet

Practice whenever and wherever you have a chance. The practice can take as little as one minute. In fact, any moment you catch yourself taking shallow breaths, try to take one or two long, deep breaths. When you exhale slowly, your heart rate slows and your body relaxes. When you begin to master the technique of lengthening your breath, keep your fingers on your neck pulse and notice that your heart slows down considerably during your exhalation.

Before you practice lengthening the breath, get a baseline of how you are breathing now. Take one minute to count the number of breaths you take normally without trying to slow or lengthen your breath. When I first started, I was taking nine breaths per minute. After three weeks I was able to get to four BPM and it came much more naturally.

In the practice below, called belly breathing, we use a three:five second ratio between inhaling and exhaling. Use this as a guideline, but it is more important to follow your own body.

11.2 Week two exercises: Belly breathing and flexibility

11.2a Belly breathing

The easiest way to learn how to breathe from your belly is to lay flat on the floor in a supine position. The floor is best because the firmness will make it easier for you to feel your lungs and ribs expanding and contracting with each breath. Use a yoga mat if needed.

1. Begin lying flat on the floor. (If you are not able to lie down, then sit or stand in a comfortable, relaxed position.)

2. Relax your body and place a hand over your belly button and the other hand just below your chest at the top of your abs.

3. Notice how you are breathing. Notice the depth and pace of your breathing. Is your breath coming only to your throat? Your chest? Is your stomach expanding at all?

4. Once you've established where your breath is, try to deepen it by gently expanding your belly with your next inhalation. It helps to first expel as much air as you can. Try to empty your lungs and draw in the air gently and slowly through your nostrils. Notice your hand rising as you inhale.

5. In addition to the feedback you are getting from your hands, you can also place a stuffed animal or a pillow on your belly and observe the rise and fall as you try to deepen your breath. Exhale slowly either through your nose or your mouth. As you exhale, softly contract your abs to help push the air out. See if you can expand and raise the belly an inch or two as you progress comfortably towards deeper breaths.

6. Practice for five to ten minutes.

When you are done, reflect on how you feel. How does your mind feel? How does your body feel? Write down some of your reflections below to deepen your learning.

This practice is a great way to relax at the end of a day. If you have any lower back issues you might put some pillows under your knees or bend your knees so you are in a semi-supine position, as in Figure 18.

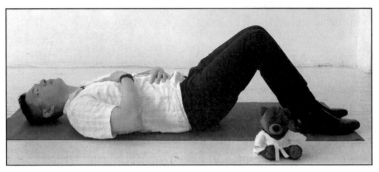

Figure 18

Benefits of Belly Breathing

Increases Body Awareness: Breath is an important window into the body. It allows us to become aware of what's going on in the body as we learned in week one. It can be an anchor that provides us feedback in terms of how we are feeling about a situation. As you breathe, are there certain areas that seem stuck or stiff?

Helps Regulate Difficult Emotions: Consciously regulating and lengthening the breath can be a powerful tool for coping with difficult emotions like anger, anxiety, depression, and stress.

Deepens Stretches: The coordination of breathing with stretching will enable you to intensify and deepen stretches so you can let go of tension and increase the body's range of motion.

Improves Heart Health: Lengthening the breath consciously can lower blood pressure and heart rate, which helps reduce stress throughout your day.

Helps Create Calm and Relaxation: Taking long and deep breaths helps relax all the various systems in the body including the nervous system, the muscular system, and the neurological system. Breathing deeply and slowly is an important method for reducing tension and stress held in the body.

11.2b Flexibility

Building on what was learned from body awareness, this week participants learn flexibility MOVEs that will help increase their range of motion, mobility, and reduce soreness and stiffness. Flexibility MOVEs are particularly important for the office worker who spends a majority of the day in a chair. As discussed in week three, sitting puts the body in an unhealthy position that shortens postural muscles and lengthens movement muscles leading to imbalances throughout the body. Flexibility MOVEs are an important part of the solution for undoing the negative effects of sitting.

It is recommended that flexibility MOVEs be done daily. Out of the total MOVEs per day (MPD) 20 to 50 percent should be flexibility MOVEs. Participants can learn a series of flexibility MOVEs that easily fit into their day, spending only one to two minutes each time. Each week they can build on previous exercises and eventually be able to combine them to create a longer flexibility routines that they can do for 10 to 20 minutes perhaps at the end of the day to stretch and relax the entire body.

Stretching, particularly static stretching, has been a staple of traditional exercise whether as a part of warm-up or cool down or both. Static stretching involves stretching a muscle to its maximum length for 20 to 30 seconds. For a long time, this method was assumed to be the best way to warm up before physical activity. Researchers are challenging this view. Studies show:

1. Static stretching before exercise reduces the performances of runners by making their strides less economical.

2. Static stretching can reduce strength by 30 percent.

3. Static stretching did not reduce the incidence of injury across large groups.

4. *Dynamic* stretching improves strength, endurance, agility, power, oxygen uptake, and coordination.

The physical goals of flexibility MOVEs are to increase muscle and tendon suppleness, increase blood flow throughout the body, increase body temperature, and improve range of motion and coordination.

When we think of stretching typically we think about holding a static (no movement) position and putting weight into a certain area of the body (e.g., putting your foot on a bench and reaching with your hand to stretch the hamstring). Passively stretching this way without conscious muscle engagement is not recommended. By stretching the joints and ligaments without muscle engagement, you put your body at risk for injury. While stretching may help muscles and joints become more flexible and loose, it also makes them less able to spring into action. Think of an overused elastic band.

To ensure that you are stretching your muscles with muscle engagement and not just passively extending your muscles and joints, focus on contracting the muscles opposite to the area being stretched. For example in a forward bend you will contract your quadriceps muscles to engage the hamstrings fully in the stretch. This is also why we bend and straighten our legs three times while doing mountain bends (See Figure 19). This would be considered dynamic stretching, but once you get the hang of it you can engage your quadriceps in connection to your hamstrings easily in a static stretch as well.

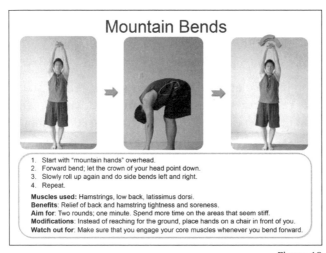

Figure 19

Here are our guiding principles when it comes to flexibility training:

1. Use dynamic stretching (e.g., standing twist, arm swings) over static stretching as a warm-up before exercise. You want to try to take your muscles through the full range of motion possible; starting slowly and then increasing speed and intensity over time.

2. Static stretching is not done with leverage or weight alone (where muscles are passively engaged). Instead we encourage the use of muscle contraction to push and stretch. This way muscles, ligaments, fascia, and joints stretch and lengthen together and injuries are avoided. For example if you are in forward bend

and are stretching your hamstrings, you will want to contract your quadriceps to go deeper into the hamstring stretch rather than using the weight of your upper body alone to intensify the hamstring stretch.

3. Generally, use static stretch with postural muscles (e.g., hamstrings, hip flexors, chest) and dynamic stretches with movement muscles (e.g., shoulders, mid-back, glutes). Stretch what shortens and move what needs to be moved. (See Week Three for review.)

4. Agonist and antagonist muscles (essentially muscles that work together) should be stretched together. An example of this is stretching your hamstrings (back of legs) and then your quadriceps (front of thighs).

5. Remember to breathe. Imagine the area you are stretching expanding and lengthening when you inhale, and relaxing and shortening when you exhale.

As we do more flexibility exercises, I encourage you to practice the lessons of body awareness with flexibility. Flexibility MOVEs are a perfect way to practice body awareness through movement.

1. Before beginning any MOVE break, create a habit of asking yourself how you are feeling, then take stock and notice how those feelings manifest in the body. Use your breath to tune in and scan internal feelings and physical sensations. The breath will help you target and release certain existing areas of tension.

2. During the flexibility MOVE breaks, remember to integrate the practices of listening to the body, lengthening the breathing, and mindfulness practices as well as healthy positions. Here are some questions you might use:

   • Where do I feel tension? Is this tension necessary?

   • How is my breathing? Can I deepen and lengthen my breath?

   • How is my position? Are my feet and knees aligned? Is my core engaged? Is my body in balance?

   As you are doing your MOVE break, listen to negative thoughts that may come up as resistance.

   "I'm not doing this right."

   "I'm too busy, I shouldn't be doing this."

"I look silly."

Notice these thoughts. Don't try to fight or change them. Focus on your will and your want, which might be you wanting to relax and stretch the body so you can feel and work better.

3. After the MOVE break, remember to reflect and reinforce your efforts. Ask yourself about the impact moving had on your mind and body. Take a few seconds to notice if you feel different or better either mentally or physically. Noticing the positive benefits of taking a break will help strengthen the habits. You could also ask, "Was that the exercise/break that I needed or would something else have been better?" Reflecting in this way will help you learn which MOVEs are the best fit in different situations.

One of the reasons why many people become unaware of the soreness, stiffness, and pain they experience from sitting is they haven't learned a way to address it. So what starts off as soreness and stiffness goes below the surface of awareness until it becomes chronic, debilitating back pain or a herniated disc. Asking reflective questions is important to create a stronger bridge between mind and body. These internal reflections and experiences are more important that any gadget in helping you create body awareness and the mind/body connection.

Working on flexibility helps maintain mobility and range of motion of muscles, joints, and ligaments well into the later stages of life. The next three weeks of the program will focus on using flexibility; however, we will also continue to learn and practice MOVEs from the other categories of body awareness, strength, core/balance, and cardio.

Benefits of flexibility moves:

- Keep the body loose and limber and reduce soreness and stiffness
- Help create relaxation and calmness throughout the body
- Reverse effects of sitting
- Improve and maintain range of motion over the long term
- Prevent injury
- Help you feel centered and grounded throughout your day
- Reduce tension
- Feel good!

11.3 Week two practice

Continue to use the scheduled triggers from week one, and add one feeling/physical sensation trigger.

Think about some of the feelings and physical sensations you noticed last week when you practiced the body awareness exercises. Pick one feeling/physical sensation trigger so that whenever you feel it you'll use it as a signal to take a MOVE break.

Try to aim for four to five MOVE breaks per day (MPDs) or pick a goal that is challenging and realistic for you. You can focus a majority of your MOVEs on the flexibility exercises (with some of them being body awareness as well) and begin to incorporate what you learned from week one regarding body awareness into the Flexibility moves.

There are eight different flexibility exercises. You can try to do half of them on one day and the other half the next day; alternating in this way for the week. Familiarize yourself with all the exercises.

Alternatively, you can do all eight exercises every day by taking two-minute-long MOVE breaks and doing one exercise for a minute and then trying another in the second minute.

The important thing is to try all of the flexibility MOVEs and learn how each one benefits the body. Once you are familiar with all the exercises you can pick the ones that will address your need in the moment.

Consult Exercise 11 and see if you have a goal to reduce stiffness, pain, or soreness. Connect this goal to the MOVEs you will do this week and use either the ThinkMOVE app or the daily journal from the download kit to record your experience and reflections. See Figures 20–27 for exercises you can try.

Try the belly breathing exercise two to three times this week and practice becoming aware of your breathing throughout the day.

When you practice flexibility moves, try to remember to breathe consciously and deeply in order to soften into the stretch and release any excessive tension.

TEAM MOVE: In your teams or with a colleague/trusted friend, share what your feeling-based trigger is for this week. Discuss why you picked this trigger and what you hope to experience from doing a MOVE break in response to it.

Goals people might have for improving flexibility include:
(Place a checkmark beside the goals that are important to you.)

	Reduced muscle soreness and/or stiffness
	Increased range of motion
	Increased mindfulness; the ability to be present and focused
	Reduced muscle pain and tension
	Increased body control; the ability to hold difficult position for longer time
	Increased body awareness through use of stretching as a method of self-care/self-awareness
	Increased moments of calmness and relaxation
	Other:

Finally, plan and strategize together any barriers (e.g., travel, workload) that may get in the way of you doing MOVE breaks this week. What strategies could you use on your own? What strategies could the team use collectively to overcome barriers?

12. Week Three: Balance and Healthy Positions

Objectives for week three: Balance and healthy positions.

- Learn about the benefits of balance MOVEs
- Learn how to create healthy positions so that you can reduce aches and pains
- Learn a series of balance moves and improve stabilizing muscles
- Use behavioral triggers as a way of triggering MOVE breaks
- Practice doing balance MOVEs together as a team and supporting each other

12.1 Week three lesson

Balance is not something to which many of us devote time and energy. Often we are caught up in trying to get strong or fitter so we do strength or cardio workouts. Whether we train it or not, we use balance all the time. Whenever we walk, go up stairs, get in our cars, and are sitting or

Standing Twist

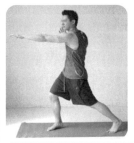

1. Twist your torso left to right continuously, shifting your head in line with your body.
2. Lift one foot off the ground (the one you are turning away from) and stretch your hip flexors (where your quad inserts into your hip) as you twist.

Muscles used: Whole body; specifically torso and upper and lower back.
Benefits: This exercise loosens the whole body. Excellent after sitting for a long time.
Aim for: One minute.
Modifications: Vary the movement of the arms to stimulate other areas of the back.
Watch out for: The upper body bending. The upper body should always be straight.

Figure 20

Warrior 1

1. Place feet in a lunge position.
2. Ensure that both feet are facing forward.
3. Reach up with your hands towards the sky.
4. You should feel a nice stretch in your hip flexor.
5. Do one side, then switch feet after 30 seconds.

Muscles used: Legs primarily, but also core.
Benefits: Stretches the hip flexor and quadriceps; works on balance.
Aim for: Do 30 seconds on each side; try to breathe deeply three times on each side.
Modifications: Narrow the foot stance to make it easier; widen for more challenge.

Figure 21

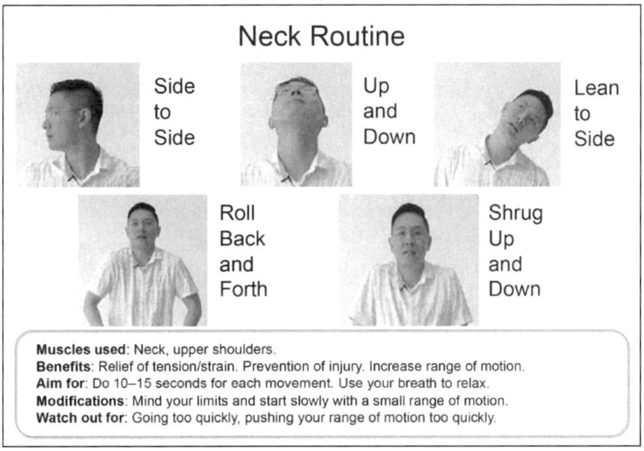

Neck Routine

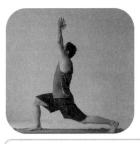

Side to Side

Up and Down

Lean to Side

Roll Back and Forth

Shrug Up and Down

Muscles used: Neck, upper shoulders.
Benefits: Relief of tension/strain. Prevention of injury. Increase range of motion.
Aim for: Do 10–15 seconds for each movement. Use your breath to relax.
Modifications: Mind your limits and start slowly with a small range of motion.
Watch out for: Going too quickly, pushing your range of motion too quickly.

Figure 22

Chair Glutes

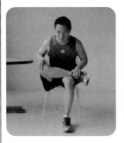

1. Sit with your bum well supported by the chair (your thighs mostly off the chair), and your back straight.
2. Cross your left leg so that the ankle rests on top of your right leg. Place your hands on your foot and knee of the left leg, press down gently, and lean forward with your back straight.

Muscles used: Glutes (your butt); hips.
Benefits: This is an exercise you can use in meetings. It counters the impact of sitting.
Aim for: Try 15-30 seconds on each side.
Modifications: An alternative version done from the floor may be safer for some.

Figure 23

Chair Hamstring Stretch

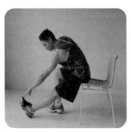

1. Sit with your bum well supported by the chair (your thighs mostly off the chair) and your back straight.
2. Bend the right leg and straighten the left leg in front of you. Bend the left foot so the toes are curling towards the left knee stretching the left hamstring.
3. You can lean forward to increase the intensity of the stretch.

Muscles used: Hamstrings.
Benefits: Loosens the hamstrings which tighten from sitting for long periods.
Aim for: Try 15-30 seconds for each leg.
Modifications: Simple leg stretch for light intensity. Reach with your hand and flex the toe back for more intensity.
Watch out for: You should experience pull but not pain. Back off if you feel pain.

Figure 24

Arm Swings

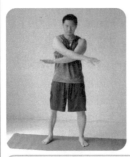

1. Swing your arms across your chest and then wide, expanding and reaching back as far as you can.
2. As your arms go back open up the chest and point your hands with thumbs point up.
3. Alternate which arm is on top each repetition.

Muscles used: Chest, shoulders, and arms.
Benefits: Opens up the chest which helps reverse the impact of rounded shoulders
Aim for: Do 20 to 30 repetitions or one minute.
Modifications: This is a dynamic stretch. You could switch to static hold using the wall.
Watch out for: Flailing the arms carelessly. Start slowly and increase speed gradually.

Figure 25

standing, we are constantly negotiating our balance between our feet and between the muscles at the front of our bodies and the back.

Poor posture is the result of improper balance between parts of the body. You can notice this whenever you end up slouched over your keyboard at work.

Practicing balance will help you learn to listen deeply to the various parts of your body as they coordinate and work together to keep you in balance. From your feet all the way to the top of your head, every muscle in the body is involved with maintaining balance. When you practice balance, focus on listening to your body and watching the micro-movements that take place. Use your breath as an anchor to let go of any unnecessary tension (of course some tension is necessary, otherwise you'd be a limp noodle).

Psychologically, balance MOVEs help teach us to not take ourselves so seriously and instead to be playful, to surrender to the moment, and be light. They require a balance between effort and effortlessness.

Balance requires honest effort and if we don't try our best we quickly fall out of balance. We must listen and be present to the moment and our body in space if we are to be in balance. This week's moves will help you improve your focus as well as regulating emotions whenever you fall out of position and have to try again.

Benefits of balance:

- Improve daily functioning (including posture)
- Prevent injury by improving posture and holding healthier positions throughout your day
- Improve focus/concentration by staying in the present moment and focusing on one thing at time
- Cultivate playfulness (have fun!)
- Improve frustration tolerance

For most, the word "posture" conjures up images of rigidity, like a soldier standing at attention with shoulders pulled back, chest out, stomach tucked in, and legs pressed together. Posture may also bring up images of stillness and being frozen like a statue. In reality, the body is never perfectly still and if you are breathing properly (diaphragmatic breathing as we discussed) the body is in constant motion by the expansion of your lungs and the movement of your stomach, chest, and shoulders, even while you are sitting or standing.

Instead of the word posture, a more appropriate word for the human frame would be the word position(s). Only telephone poles maintain perfect posture. It is unrealistic and unhealthy to expect our bodies to hold up postures all day as if we were statues. By moving away from the word posture, I hope to encourage you to change positions constantly throughout the day and practice moving in more effective and efficient ways.

Understanding some fundamental principles of healthy positions for standing, sitting, walking, and exercise can help improve overall functioning, feelings of health and vitality, prevent injury, and prolong the life of muscles, bones, and ligaments.

Poor positions are a result of a body being trained by thousands of hours of sitting. Poor positions are a learned behavior that begin when children reach school age. Their bodies get caged into chairs and behind desks and they are taught to sit still and not fidget. It takes some time and effort to unschool our sedentary physical education and learn how to use our bodies intelligently so that we are moving in dynamic and healthy ways.

Now that we have developed some skills of awareness and listening to the body (week one), and breathing (week two), we can integrate these skills to use healthier positions when we sit, stand, move, or exercise.

As you become aware of your position, don't try to move yourself into the "correct" posture. The aim is freeing the body, not imprisoning it further. Instead, focus first on pausing and becoming aware of what you are doing and how you are using your body. By approaching your body in a relaxed way (not forcing) you can naturally move your body into a healthier position.

Postural Muscles & Movement Muscles

Standing up like a soldier with your head craned back and your chest puffed is unhealthy for two reasons. First, the head is pulled back causing strain in the neck. The shoulder blades slightly winged and the lower back overarched result in a condition called lordosis. This creates excessive muscle tension, particularly in the low back that most people can only hold for a few minutes before returning to a slouched, limp noodle position!

Second, the body consists of postural and movement muscles. The postural muscles are designed to be active for longer periods than movement muscles. These muscles enable us to hold the body up while we sit and stand. However, being stuck in any fixed position for long periods will lead to fatigue and muscle strain. When we command ourselves to "stand up straight! Don't slouch!" for hours and hours, we overwork the postural muscles and create unnecessary tension throughout the body.

The problem isn't that we are not using our postural muscles enough. In fact, due to prolonged sitting, the opposite is true: We are relying on them too much and in really bad positions. Excessive use of postural muscles creates weaknesses in our movement-based muscles (also called phasic muscles). This results in imbalances throughout the entire musculoskeletal system.

As the name implies, movement muscles are designed for movement and are not designed to hold the body in a "correct posture" for an entire day. When these muscles are held chronically in a fixed position (i.e., sitting), it leads to fatigue, pain, stiffness, and sometimes injury.

Because most people maintain poor posture while sitting or standing, your low back, mid back, and upper shoulder muscles (postural muscles) are working hard to keep your face from crashing into the keyboard while your abs, glutes, and chest (movement muscles) are mostly shut off. This lack of muscle activation leads to muscle atrophy which creates further imbalances in the body. This repeated pattern makes it more and more difficult to maintain healthy positions.

Movement-based muscles ought to play an important role in aiding and supporting postural muscles in holding the body in healthy, well-balanced positions. For example, your low back can be aided by some abdominal activation (muscle contraction) to create balance and to maintain a healthy position. After 20 minutes or even an hour, even if you are balancing well, the muscles get tired from overuse and therefore I recommend that you give your muscles regular breaks from being in fixed positions (i.e., changing the position or moving once every 20 minutes).

If there is tension and strain in the body, we can use MOVE breaks to engage movement (phasic) muscles to help relieve the tension. By doing this, movement muscles are strengthened, loosened, and lengthened. This helps the postural muscles relax and coordinate with the movement muscles more efficiently. The combination of engaging postural and movement muscles together and taking regular breaks from stationary

Exercise 12
How Are You Using Your Body Right Now?

Take a moment to notice the position of your body right now, whether you are sitting or standing. Remember there this is no single correct posture that you are expected to maintain. From here you can make choices that might help you feel better and healthier.

BREATHING: How are you breathing right now? Deep or shallow?

FEET: In what position are your feet? Are they crossed over each other or wrapped around the chair? In what position are your legs? Do you like to cross your legs?

ABS: Are your abs engaged at all? Is your low back tight/rounded? Are you sitting more on one bum cheek than the other?

SHOULDERS: Are your shoulders positioned inward? Rolled back? Is your upper shoulder area tight? Are your shoulders held up towards your ears?

HEAD: Is your head tilted upwards or downwards? Do you tend to lean your head more to one side than the other? Where does your gaze fall?

Write down your observations below:
BREATHING:
_____
_____
_____

FEET:
_____
_____
_____

ABS:
_____
_____

SHOULDERS:
_____
_____
_____

HEAD:
_____
_____
_____

positions results in the body being more capable of holding healthier positions. A breakdown of postural muscles and movement muscles is in Figure 26.

12.2 Week three exercises

The idea of improving posture is a complex, challenging, and important task. It is unrealistic to think that the task will be completed just

Postural (Tonic) Muscles	Movement (Phasic) Muscles
Characteristics: • Generally flexor (bend) or postural muscles • Tendency to tightness or shortening (therefore it is good to stretch these) • Easily activated and fatigue quickly; less likely to atrophy • Less fragile • Typically one-joint muscles	**Characteristics:** • Generally extensor (straighten) muscles • Tendency towards weakness or lengthening (therefore it is good to strengthen these) • Delayed activation, weak • More likely to atrophy • More fragile • Typically two-joint muscles
KEY IDEA: If movement muscles are underused in relation to postural muscles, postural muscles will get overused and fatigued creating weakness in the movement muscles and imbalances in the body	
NEEDS: Prolonged sitting leads to muscle imbalance that **shorten** POSTURAL muscles. Therefore these muscles would benefit from massage, stretching and rest	**NEEDS:** Prolonged sitting leads to weakness of the following MOVEMENT muscles. This occurs because they are maintained in a **lengthened** position for long periods and are underutilized while sitting. These muscles would benefit from strengthening and some stretching particularly dynamic stretching
List of Postural Muscles • Gastroc-Soleus (calves) • Hip Adductors • Hamstrings • Rectus Femoris (one of the quadriceps part of hip flexor) • Iliopsoas (one of hip flexors) • Tensor Fascia Lata (hip flexors) • Piriformis (part of butt muscles) • Erector-Spinae (thoraco-lumbar) (Lumbar spine extensors) • Suboccipital muscles (muscles at base of spine) • Quadratus Lumborum (low back muscle) • Pectoralis Major and Minor (Chest) • Latissimus Dorsi (back muscles) • Upper Trapezius (upper shoulders) • Levator Scapulae (back and side of neck, lifts scapula) • Scalenes (side of neck at front) • Sternocleidomastoid (muscles at side of neck)	**List of Movement Muscles** • Deltoids (shoulder) • Triceps (back of arms) • Peroneals (muscles in calves for ankle stability) • Tibialis Anterior (muscle in front of shin bone) • Vastus Medialis (teardrop part of quadricep) • Vastus Lateralis (outside part of quadricep) • Gluteus Maximus (butt muscles) • Gluteus Medius (small butt muscle) • Transversus Abdominus • Multifidus (muscles along the spine) • Rectus Abominus (abs) • Abdominal Obliques (obliques) • Serratus Anterior (serratus) involved in breathing • Rhomboids (between shoulder blades and the mid back) • Lower and Middle Trapezius (upper shoulders) • Deep neck flexors (front of neck)
The Muscle Groups in Layperson's Terms (Listed in Order of Their Pairings)	
• Middle of thigh (connected to hip) • Low back muscles • Chest • Back and side of neck	• Outer and inner thigh • Abdominals and butt muscles • Middle of back • Front of neck

Figure 26

by reading about it. However, it is our hope that this information has planted the seed for some positive changes and with practice and awareness you will experience less muscle tension and prevent injury, back pain, and premature aging.

The main message here is not to search for a better way to be still, frozen, or rigid, which is the whole problem of being sedentary. Instead it is to recognize the body's need for movement and to move in healthy positions while sitting, standing, or moving.

What is important to remember is that the body is not designed to be in any single position for prolonged periods of time. Sitting happens to be the main problematic position we engage. This is why we recommend changing positions every 20 minutes or taking a MOVE break once every 20 minutes. Poor posture can become a useful behavioral trigger that signals, "it's time to MOVE!" That being said we will review how to stand in a healthy body position in the next section.

In the healthy position exercises below, we review the ways to engage both postural and movement muscles together in order to maintain optimal stationary positions. MOVE breaks allow you to engage movement muscles that are underused while you are in a stationary position.

Here is a comprehensive review of the problems associated with prolonged sitting; particularly sitting in unhealthy positions, in Figure 27.

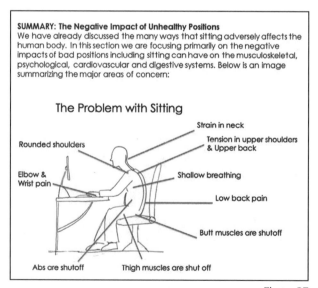

SUMMARY: The Negative Impact of Unhealthy Positions
We have already discussed the many ways that sitting adversely affects the human body. In this section we are focusing primarily on the negative impacts of bad positions including sitting can have on the musculoskeletal, psychological, cardiovascular and digestive systems. Below is an image summarizing the major areas of concern:

The Problem with Sitting

Strain in neck

Tension in upper shoulders & Upper back

Rounded shoulders

Elbow & Wrist pain

Shallow breathing

Low back pain

Butt muscles are shutoff

Abs are shutoff

Thigh muscles are shut off

Figure 27

Healthy Standing Position (HSP)

Understanding the many muscle groups that comprise the body as well as the different characteristics of postural (tonic) compared to movement (phasic) muscles helps us appreciate the complexity of the human body. When it comes to creating healthy body positions, it's not simply a matter of holding static positions well, but coordinating between these muscle groups and giving the movement muscles a chance to move with periodic breaks. Unhealthy positions overwork postural muscles and create poor or weak positions, which look like: head too far forward or back, rounded back and shoulders, excessive arch or rounding in low back, hips too far forward or back, and poor foot and knee alignment leading to weak ankle stability.

A healthy standing position requires balancing weight distribution and muscle activation throughout the body. Figure 28 shows some examples of unhealthy standing positions. Figure 29 lists the major checkpoints for healthy positions. These guiding principles can help you enhance your body's position whatever you are doing.

Standing is the best stationary position to practice from because you need to balance the entire weight of your body on your feet. When you are sitting or lying down, the chair or the bed does a lot of the work for you so you lose a lot of sensory feedback about what the postural and movement muscles are doing. By first learning the principles of healthy positions while standing, you will be able to generalize

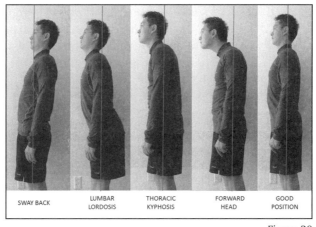

Figure 28

The Negative Impacts of Unhealthy Positions

Musculoskeletal	Psychological	Digestive	Cardio	Others
Muscle and bone atrophy	Poor posture can lead to low mood (increase in depression) and low energy	Lowered insulin sensitivity	Increased blood pressure and cholesterol	Slowed brain function; less oxygen and blood circulation to the brain
No electrical activity in legs and movement muscles of body		Increased glucose in blood	Increased risk for cardiac disease	
	Gives an appearance of weakness and low confidence	Fewer fat burning enzymes		Less effective immune system
Low back pain; shortening and tightening of muscles and ligaments		Poor digestion due to lack of diaphragmatic breathing	Poor circulation in legs (i.e., varicose veins and blood clots)	Increased risk of cancer (due to increases in insulin and fewer natural antioxidants)
	Lowers self-confidence			
C spine creating an inflexible spine	Poor self-image		Lowered aerobic capacity	
Tight hip flexors; limp glutes; weak abs; weak quadriceps	Reduced focus and mental alertness			Shallow breathing; lower oxygen absorption
	Less energy			
Strained neck	Shallow breathing leads to stress on the nervous system			
Increased risk for disk damage				
Can lead to muscle fatigue and strain (later pain)	The heart and lungs need to work harder			

Figure 29

these principles more easily to healthier sitting, walking, and other movement patterns. The acronym FASH is a tool that can help you remember the major checkpoints: Feet, Abs, Shoulders, and Head.

The first step in moving towards healthier positions is to reduce excessive tension, specifically with postural muscle activation. Often when people notice their poor posture or they are prompted by someone to fix their posture, they will throw their shoulders back and over-arch their lower back and stick out their chest. As we have discussed, this is not a healthy position. Instead, you can start by relaxing and becoming aware of what you are doing with your body and by breathing. Take a moment to notice the areas of tension that usually occur in the calves, hamstrings, lower back, chest, upper back, upper shoulders, and neck, and relaxing them.

Once you have put your body in a state of relaxed awareness and the overactive postural muscles have relaxed, some muscle activation in the phasic muscles (e.g., abs, glutes, midback, external rotators of shoulder) will help balance the body's position. For example, engaging the lower abs to support the low back and engaging the mid back (rhomboids) to open and widen the chest.

HEALTHY STANDING POSITION		
AREA	WHAT TO DO	EXERCISE
FEET	First, draw your hands pointed as guns with your index fingers pointing down from the middle of your thighs. Try to line up the center of your hips with the center of your thighs, then your knees down to your feet. Second, notice the position of your feet. Make sure they are facing forward (second toe pointing forward) and be aware of the weight distribution between each foot and leg. Try to balance yourself equally on each foot and on all **three** pods of each foot. Make sure your arches are activated and not collapsed. Make sure your knees are facing forward. Let your knees bend directly over your feet and not to the side or inwards to your centerline. Aim to line up your knees with your second toe. Imagine the screwdriver effect (as knees rotate externally your feet will get more connected to the ground). Keep the knees slightly bent; not locked out.	Arch doming; Balancing MOVEs to increase strength and endurance in feet. **Three Pods of Foot** Squats; Single leg squats to improve strength in feet and knees
ABS & PELVIS	Pelvis is rolled forward or back so the bowl is flat; not tipping backwards or forwards; nor tipping to the left or right. Engage the lower abs at 20% to help tip the bowl backwards so it is properly balanced and the hip flexors are lengthened.	Strengthen the abdominals; Stretch the low back; Strengthen the glutes; Stretch the hamstrings; Stretch the hip flexors
SHOULDERS	Roll shoulders back and down. Both shoulders should be relaxed and down and equal level from left to right. Shoulder blades moved towards each other with rhomboids (mid back muscles) engaged. Chest should be open and lengthened allowing natural breath to expand the chest. Arms externally rotated with thumbs out.	Back flyes; bent over rows.
HEAD	Head back; forward and up; Ears should be over shoulders Being mindful not to just lean the head back and putting excessive strain on the neck but engage the deep neck flexors to position the head back. Neck is a neutral position; well balanced. Eye gaze is at the horizon.	Chin tucks; Neck routine

Figure 30

Three Exercises: Healthy Standing Position and Wiggling

Healthy Standing Position (B-FASH)

This exercise will help you put your entire body into a healthy standing position. First take a natural standing position without trying to fix or correct anything. As you move towards awareness of your body's position don't do anything or make any effort to move yourself into a better position. What we will practice today is the skill of allowing the healthier position to occur naturally by freeing the body of unnecessary tension.

1. **BREATHE**: Begin by taking three deep breaths. Imagine your whole body is a lung. Breathing in and expanding, stretching, lengthening and then exhaling relaxing, contracting, shortening. Let your whole body breathe. As you do this, see if you can allow your spine, neck to lengthen (pause), your stomach and ribs to expand, lengthen, and constrict with the inhalation and exhalation. (pause) Notice the rise and fall of your chest as you take in deep nourishing breaths.

2. **FEET**: Next, pay attention to your feet. Look down and try to position your feet so they are facing forward and in line with your hips and your knees. Notice how the weight is distributed between them. Is your weight leaned more heavily to one side? Feel if you can let your weight be shared equally between your feet. Pay attention also to the position your feet are in, facing forward and in line with your knees. Notice any unnecessary tension that may exist in your legs and see if you can relax and let your legs and the bones of within them hold you upright.

3. **ABS**: Next, pay attention to your abdominals and your low back. Your trunk. See if you are over arching your low back and creating tension there. Most people over arch their low backs and carry a lot of tension here. You can use your hands to feel if this is the case. Imagine your waist band is the tip of a bowl, a pelvic bowl. Tip your pelvic bowl forward and then backwards (pause) then use deep belly breathing to lighten the tension there and imagine creating space between the vertebrae and each column extending upwards lightly, effortlessly. Allow your body to find the neutral position of your spine. Relax the back as much as you can while maintaining an upright position. Imagine the breath creating space between the muscle fibers and lengthening them. If you notice that you are able to reduce the tension in the low back you can complete this section by tightening your lower abs slightly. Continue to breath deeply and feel how tightening the abs can further relieve the tension in the low back and help tip the pelvic bowl into a balanced position

4. **SHOULDERS**: Next focus on your shoulder area and chest and back area. Let the breathing expand the chest open and bring the shoulders back and down naturally. As you breath to relax the shoulders and the upper trapezius, which are often sore from excessive tension. Let your shoulders drop and relax with your next exhalation (pause). Let the shoulders roll back and down so that they are of equal level. Bring your shoulders blades together so your middle back is engaged slightly. Breathe. With your arms by your side rotate them externally so your palms face forward and your thumbs are out.

5. **HEAD**: Let your head move back if you tend to lurch your head forward. Tuck your chin in an lengthen the back of your neck slightly. Move your head so your ears fall directly over your shoulders. Be mindful not to just lean the head back putting excessive strain on the neck but to engage deep neck flexors to position the head back. Keep the neck in a neutral relaxed position; well balanced from left to right and forward and back. Keep your eye gaze at the horizon

Improving your standing position will take time and practice. Be patient with yourself. There may be a particular area that is particularly relevant for you. Perhaps you tend to overarch your low back. You might then focus on the abdominal/low back area whenever you practice healthy standing if the rest of your positioning is fine.

Wiggling

This is a simple practice to help you increase your awareness of your body through movement. It will also help you reduce tension and increase relaxation.

1. VISUALIZE A BAMBOO TREE. Begin by just standing up and imagining yourself as a bamboo tree or any young tree that you've seen whose branches bend easily with the wind. Move yourself out of being a stiff telephone pole for a while. Imagine a gentle wind pushing you forward and back and like an Olympic swimmer who prepares himself or herself before the start of a race let your limbs just wiggle. Remember a time when you may have been out, in nature, a park, or the woods, and that so much of life wiggles, shakes, moves. See and feel the trees, bushes, the branches, the flowers: All these things wiggle, they bend, and flex, and move naturally. We forget this natural state of movement when we find ourselves stuck in square buildings, behind square desks, conforming our bodies to rigid 90-degree angles like the structures that house us.

2. START TO WIGGLE. So wiggle your toes and fingers. Wiggle your legs, bending your knees, let your hips move about forward and back and in circles, experiment with all the varieties of movement your body can express. Raise your hands up as far as they will go, then to the side and back wiggling your fingers. Notice the way your back and shoulders join the dance when you move your arms about. You may feel the hard armor of stiffness loosening as you wiggle and shake off the cobwebs. In the same way with your hands play with the movement of legs, raise a knee towards your waist, flex your foot back towards your butt. Swing your leg forward and back and then side to side, being aware and attentive to your balance; stay centered and grounded.

3. WIGGLE YOUR LOW BACK. Give some attention to your back particularly your low back which gets stuck in the cage of a chair for so many hours. Let it shift and move and wiggle about. Let the tension release with each wiggle, practicing breathing into the space between the movement and let relaxation take the place of tension.

4. NECK. Give some attention and wiggle time to your neck, notice all the varieties of angles in which it can move, turning your head in all directions so it can look up and down to the sides and in circles. What a unique gift our neck gives us.

Figure 30 — Continued

5. HEAD/FACE. Now turn your attention to your face and let your eyes move about and your cheeks and mouth wiggle about and your brow wiggle about. Let your whole body wake up through movement and let yourself become aware of the feelings and sensations that this gift of wiggle can give you.

"The idea is that flowing water never goes stale, so just keep on flowing."

— Bruce Lee

This is practice that will help relieve tension and help loosen the body. You can practice it anytime; mornings and before bed are excellent times. It may seem strange at first to move the body in this way, but give it a try and let yourself experience the benefits of these small and gentle movements on the body. People naturally engage in this wiggling when they stretch their shoulders and move their necks after long periods of sitting. This practice encourages you to do the same for the rest of the body.

Figure 30 — Continued

Staying in any position, whether standing, sitting, or walking for extended periods of time, will create strain, tension and fatigue in the body. This is why it is recommended that people take breaks and change positions every 20 minutes. It could be as simple as going from sitting to standing or shifting your position in your chair if you need to remain seated.

These are the moves for this week:

1. Plank
2. Captain stance
3. Standing Superman
4. Single leg squat
5. Desk reptile

12.3 Week three practice

Continue to use the scheduling feeling triggers from previous weeks and add one behavioral trigger.

Think about a typical behavior that you could use to trigger a move. This might be: "When I ... , I will do a move."

Example: "When I notice poor posture, I will take a MOVE BREAK."

Try to aim for five to six MOVE breaks per day (MPDs) with at least two of the five being balance moves every day.

Balance moves require focus as you constantly negotiate your weight on one foot. There is a dance that happens with all the muscles and bones of your body. Allow yourself to be present to those micro-movements and be mindful of your breath so you can let go of any unnecessary tension that may be there. Remember FASH and keep your body in healthy positions throughout the balance exercises.

Plank

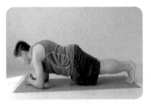

1. Press your forearms on the floor (or desk) and clasp hands as if in a prayer posture.
2. Keep your head, back, and legs aligned.
3. You can also plank from your desk. It will be easier but still effective in training your abs.

Muscles used: Core; abdominals and low back.
Benefits: One of the best ways to strengthen your core.
Aim for: Try 30 to 60 seconds or more.
Modifications: Do this move from an elevated plane (e.g., desk) or from your knees.
Watch out for: Collapsing of low back, bending neck, holding breath.

Figure 31

Captain Stance

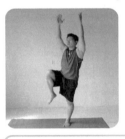

1. This is a balance move where you can practice body awareness and mindfulness.
2. Hold one leg up so the thigh is parallel to the floor with your hands pointing up towards the ceiling for 30 seconds, then switch legs for another 30 seconds.

Muscles used: Core and legs.
Benefits: This exercise challenges ankle stability and foot strength.
Aim for: Do 30 to 60 seconds on each side.
Modifications: To make it harder, close your eyes.
Watch out for: Knee/foot alignment; disengaged core; always keep your abs engaged.

Figure 32

Standing Superman

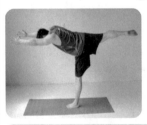

1. Starting in a standing position, lean forward with your arms outstretched and your head in a neutral position.
2. Lift one leg behind you so that there is a straight line from your raised foot all the way across your body to your fingertips.
3. You can choose to hold for a second at the top then return to standing, then alternating legs, and hold on each side for as long as you can.

Muscles used: Core and legs.
Benefits: This exercise challenges ankle stability and foot strength.
Aim for: Try 30 to 60 seconds on each side.
Modifications: To make it harder close your eyes.
Watch out for: Knee/foot alignment; disengaged core; always keep your abs engaged.

Figure 33

Single Leg Squat

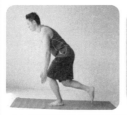

1. Put one leg up like a pink flamingo, hands on hips, or out in front of you.
2. Tap the toes of the foot that is elevated on the floor. Try not to step with the back foot unless you have to.

Muscles used: Legs, core stabilizers.
Benefits: Strengthens the leg and works on balance as well.
Aim for: Do 10–20 repetitions on each leg.
Modifications: Vary the depth of the squat or practice holding an object if needed.
Watch out for: Misalignment of the foot and knee; rounding of back.

Figure 34

Desk Reptile

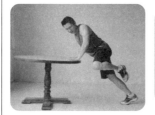

Knees come up to the side, to the outside of the elbows as you hold a desk. Alternate one knee after the other.

Muscles used: Heart, abs, obliques, legs.
Benefits: This is a dynamic movement that works the heart and abs.
Aim for: One-minute continuous movement.
Modifications: Bring the knees to the front if it is too difficult to bring them to the elbow.
Watch out for: Make sure your desk is sturdy and you have a good grip on the table.

Figure 35

Do you have a goal to reduce stiffness, pain, or soreness? Maintaining healthy positions whether you are sitting, standing, or moving will help reduce stiffness and pain particularly in the low back, but sometimes also in the shoulders and neck area.

You may also have had a goal to improve focus and cope with stress. Practicing healthier positions and balance moves will help you return to the present moment and connect with your body. Keep this in mind as you practice balance. Remember to let yourself breathe and let go of unnecessary tension.

Connect your goal to the MOVEs you will do this week and use your ThinkMOVE journal to record your experience and reflections of the MOVE breaks.

Try the healthy positions exercise of FASH at least two times each day. Pay extra attention to your positions throughout the day and be aware when you are in unhealthy positions. Use this as a trigger to move yourself into a healthier one.

Try to do two balance MOVES a day. When you practice balance moves try to remember to breathe consciously and deeply in order to stay present and release any excessive tension.

In your teams or with a colleague/trusted friend, share what your behavior-based trigger is for this week. Discuss why you picked this trigger and what you hope to experience from doing a MOVE break in response to it.

Finally, plan and strategize together any barriers (e.g., travel, workload) that may get in the way of you doing MOVE breaks this week.

Now that you've learned some of the principles of a healthy standing position, you can recognize unhealthy positions when they happen. If you have been in a fixed position for a long time, it is natural that you will drift into an unhealthy position because of fatigue. Instead of being hard on yourself, simply use this as a trigger: It's time for a MOVE break. Poor posture and unhealthy positions are habits we've learned over many years. It will take some time to learn how to move in healthy positions.

Yoga positions and flows are excellent ways to improve posture because they challenge the body to engage all muscles simultaneously through dynamic movement. Movement muscles (phasic) and postural muscles (tonic) coordinate and work together to create balance. Yoga strikes a unique balance between holding static positions and movement. This balance can create healing in the body because it trains the musculoskeletal system to fully and dynamically engage both postural muscles (to hold the body in a position) and the movement-based muscles (to transition the body from one position to the next).

13. Week Four: Strength and Stringing

Objectives for week four: Strength and stringing

- Learn about the benefits of strength MOVEs on physical and mental health

- Deepen practice of breathing and healthy positions through strength MOVEs

- Learn a series of strength moves and increase strength and muscle tone

- Use the stringing technique as a way of disrupting prolonged periods of sitting

- For the team to practice strength MOVEs at the office and have fun challenging each other

13.1 Week four lesson

The average adult male loses one pound of muscle every year after the age of 30. Strength training is important for muscle growth and preservation as well as improving bone density. By doing strength training, we slow the aging process by improving our ability to perform functional movements like carrying groceries, pushing heavy doors, and lifting up children. In connection to week three, increasing strength will help you hold your body in healthier positions (FASH) for longer.

The idea of doing strength moves at work might seem strange. Here's how they will benefit you and your team.

There are three layers of benefit in everything we do in the Think-MOVE program:

1. Physical (personal): e.g., weight loss, pain reduction, less prolonged sitting time.

2. Mental (personal): e.g., improved mood, better stress management.

3. Relational/organizational (communal): e.g., greater connection and communication.

The first two relate to personal benefits that you might experience and the third involves the experience of the organization as a group. Let's explore physical and relational benefits first and we'll address the psychological benefits in the next section.

If you are currently not doing any regular strength training, Think-MOVE is a great way to incorporate strength movements and to stimulate the musculoskeletal system. Practicing strength MOVEs through the ThinkMOVE program will help you build a foundation towards a traditional strength training program.

If you do engage in regular strength training, (statistically, you are part of a small group of only 15 percent of the population) you might think doing strength MOVEs during your day is pointless. However, there are many benefits you can still experience. Practicing strength exercises is a great way to boost energy and counteract the effects of sitting. For example, if you've had a really tough leg workout, doing lower intensity strength MOVEs can help aid the recovery process by stimulating blood flow and preventing muscle atrophy by stimulating the muscles that would otherwise be turned off during hours of sitting a day.

Also, using the ThinkMOVE system can be an opportunity to work on aspects of your strength that you don't have time for at the gym (e.g., grip strength, legs if you tend to avoid legs day, and core strength).

If you are regularly strength training, doing strength MOVES at the office can be a great way to be a leader and role model for others who are intimidated by gyms and avoid them.

You can support your coworkers who have yet to engage in strength training. Encourage them, challenge them, and coach them with what you know. They need your support, otherwise they might not feel comfortable trying something new. By having everyone participate positively, it creates a positive association to all the elements of the program that would benefit each person. By doing strength MOVEs during the day, you create a win for your body and a win for the company culture, which benefits everyone.

Doing strength MOVEs can be a great way to create connection and a culture of health and movement at your workplace. Transforming the work culture is not the job of one or a few, but for all.

Psychologically, strength MOVEs can increase confidence and focus. They have definitive beginnings and endings. Goals can be measured and progress can be measured and observed like the number of push ups completed in two minutes or holding a plank for time.

Strength moves have very clear boundaries since they are linear in their rhythm. They have very particular ways of being done including specific movement pattern, timing, beginnings, endings, and number of repetitions.

Strength MOVEs can be a great way for you to bring order into a day where you are experiencing a lot of chaos. Focus on the smooth rhythm of each repetition and the coordination with deep breaths. This can help you build confidence in general by giving you a concrete challenge to face multiple times throughout the day. Completing each Strength MOVE will give you a sense of mastery and accomplishment one minute at a time.

Benefits of strength:

- Boost energy
- Counteract the effects of sitting by increasing muscle activity and blood flow
- Improve confidence
- Improve focus and cope with stress and chaos of the day
- Improve functional movement
- Increase muscle tone
- Improve posture
- Have fun as a team and do challenges that create greater team connections
- Help break down culture barriers to movement at the workplace

13.2 Week four exercise: Stringing

No one can maintain 100 percent focus and productivity throughout an entire day. Stringing makes use of the power of movement to help you renew and recharge so you are managing your energy in a sustainable and efficient way.

Stringing combines productivity with health. By creating a set work to break ratio, you maximize your attention span by giving yourself regularly occurring breaks. The idea is to work in focused bursts of energy for a predetermined timeframe (e.g., 30 minutes) followed by a break of a set length (e.g., two minutes). This helps renew your energy for the next work phase.

If you have a job that requires you to sit for long periods (an hour or more at a time) then the stringing technique is built for you. For example, it's good for computer programmers or copywriters who need to be at their desk working throughout their day.

Using the stringing technique will help get you in a regular rhythm of MOVE breaks while also maximizing energy. See Figure 36.

Stringing is the most powerful way to integrate regular movement while also working in a focused and productive way.

Stringing acts as an anchor that helps you return to your body even though you may be immersed in your work. You'll find that even a brief moment of some deep breaths and movement will actually help recharge you because of the increased blood flow and oxygen.

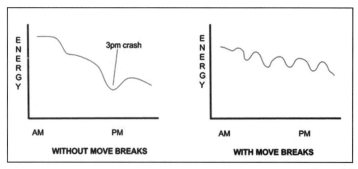

Figure 36

Some people worry they can't break their concentration even for a minute. If this is you, I would suggest trying stringing at least once and seeing how you feel. If you feel that you've lost your momentum doing the MOVE break, I would suggest doing something simple where you can still be focused on your work. Stand up and stretch your hamstrings or stand up and do some squats and allow your eyes and your mind to remain focused on your work.

Stringing could be applied as you:

- work on any writing project
- do extensive research
- prepare for a presentation
- sit for long periods as a programmer or designer
- collaborate with your team on a project that requires long meetings

Benefits of stringing:

- Improves work productivity by managing energy with regular movement breaks
- Increases mental endurance
- Enhances focus
- Uses time efficiently
- Addresses sedentary time while being productive
- Helps you break down large projects into manageable chunks

How to string (steps):

1. First establish what you'll be working on and how much time you'll be spending that day on that project(s).

2. Next break the project into manageable chunks (sub goals).

3. Set your MOVE:WORK timers in the ThinkMOVE app (ideally your move breaks are between 1 minute to 5 minutes and your work timer is between 20–40 minutes) make sure you turn on "stringing" within the ThinkMOVE app so the timers are paired.

Min:Min

Minutes for MOVE break: Minutes for WORK phase

Example: 2 minutes:30 minutes

1. Start with a MOVE and then get to work!

2. After four or five consecutive strings you might reward yourself with a longer break between 15–30 minutes. It might be time for lunch or a walk outside.

Srength exercises:

1. Squats

2. Push ups

3. Deadlifts

4. Chair isometric

5. Lunges

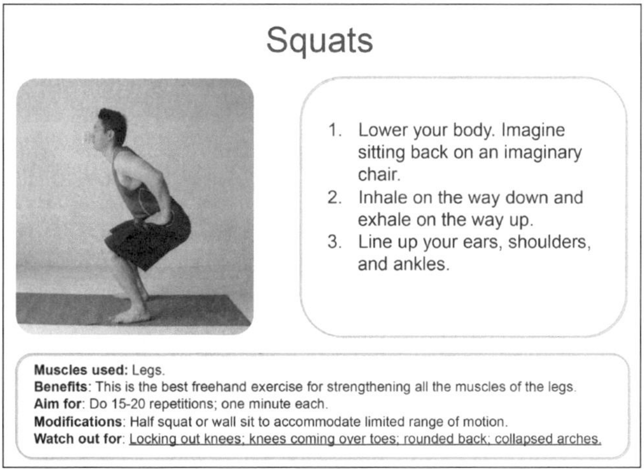

Squats

1. Lower your body. Imagine sitting back on an imaginary chair.
2. Inhale on the way down and exhale on the way up.
3. Line up your ears, shoulders, and ankles.

Muscles used: Legs.
Benefits: This is the best freehand exercise for strengthening all the muscles of the legs.
Aim for: Do 15-20 repetitions; one minute each.
Modifications: Half squat or wall sit to accommodate limited range of motion.
Watch out for: Locking out knees; knees coming over toes; rounded back; collapsed arches.

Figure 37

Push ups

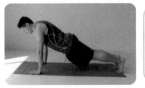

1. Take either a position from your knees or from your toes, whichever you can do for 60 seconds.
2. Try to get your arms to 90 degrees bent as you go down.
3. Keep your head in a neutral position and keep your body in alignment.

Muscles used: Chest; core.
Benefits: This is the best freehand exercise for developing upper body strength.
Aim for: As many repetitions you can do in either 30 or 60 seconds.
Modifications: Try wall or desk push ups or from the floor with knees down. Vary hand. position to target different areas of the chest. Wider for outer chest; narrow for inner chest, triceps.
Watch out for: Sagging hips, forward lurch of head, rising of shoulders.

Figure 38

(Stiff Legged) Deadlifts

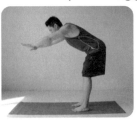

1. With your feet slightly closer than shoulder width apart, bend forward with your hands in front of you. Keep your legs as straight as possible.
2. Lower yourself as far as you can go without needing to round your back, then return.
3. Take two seconds on the way down and three to four seconds on the way up.

Muscles used: Hamstrings, abs, low back.
Benefits: Strengthens your core and increases flexibility of hamstrings.
Aim for: Do 15 to 20 repetitions or one minute.
Modifications: Only go as far down as you can while also maintaining a straight back.
Watch out for: Fatigue of the low back. Once you feel your form break, stop the exercise.

Figure 39

Chair Isometric

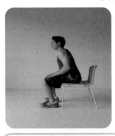

1. Sit so thighs are half off of chair.
2. Imagine pushing the ground below you with all your strength (ten seconds).
3. Rest for ten seconds.
4. Repeat two more times for one minute.

Muscles used: Legs (quadriceps, gluteus maximus).
Benefits: Stealth MOVE! Stimulate the legs during meetings.
Aim for: Three rounds of ten seconds active/ ten seconds rest.
Modifications: Extend the active time for more of a challenge.
Watch out for: Holding breath, rounding of back. Make sure to breathe and keep posture.

Figure 40

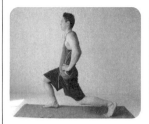

Forward Lunges

1. Step forward with your hands on your hips.
2. Both knees should be bend at 90 degrees.
3. Your torso should fall directly over your hips.
4. Keep your eyes and chin up looking at a single spot in front of you.

Muscles used: Quadriceps, hamstrings.
Benefits: Loosens the hamstrings which tighten from sitting for long periods.
Aim for: Do 10 to 12 repetitions for each leg, alternating one leg at a time.
Modifications: Do one side at a time instead of alternating legs.
Watch out for: Be mindful of any knee pain and balance issues.

Figure 41

13.3 Week four practice

Continue to use the triggers from the previous weeks and add one environmental/social trigger. An environmental trigger is a specific location that you visit regularly that would invite an opportunity to MOVE, e.g., kitchen, photocopy room, bathroom.

Think of a recurring environmental trigger at your office that would work well as a trigger for movement. For example: "Whenever I am in the kitchen microwaving my lunch, I will do some squats."

My environmental trigger for this week is:

_____

_____

_____

Whenever I find myself in _____, I will take a minute to do a MOVE break.

You might choose to use a social trigger. A social trigger is a specific and recurring social situation that would work as a trigger for movement, e.g., needing to email/call someone within your office, needing to set up an impromptu meeting, needing help on a project, feeling isolated or overwhelmed and wanting to connect with someone.

You can simply take a minute to do a MOVE break on your own or you can use the social trigger as an opportunity to do a Team MOVE with others. For example, "I want to go over the XYZ account with you. Let's meet in the boardroom and talk and do a few stretches."

My social trigger for this week is:

_____

_____

_____

Whenever _____, I will take an opportunity to do a MOVE break.

Practice the stringing technique one or two times this week. Either on your own or with your team, look at the week or day ahead and see if there are periods in your day where you'll know you'll be sitting for long periods. In your agenda, highlight those moments to practice.

You can use the ThinkMOVE app to synchronize your team so that you are taking your MOVE breaks together. Aim for six to seven MOVE breaks per day (MPDs) or pick a goal that is challenging and realistic for you. Try to do three strength MOVEs every day. Remember to keep in mind the elements of body awareness from week one as you practice strength (i.e., your breathing, position, excessive tension, etc).

Focus the rest of your MOVEs on flexibility and body awareness.

There are only five strength MOVES. Focus on one move each day aiming to do at least three sets of that move each day. For example:

MONDAY	TUESDAY	WEDNESDAY	THURSDAY	FRIDAY
3 x SQUATS	3 x DEADLIFTS	3 x PUSH UPS	3 x CHAIR	ISOMETRIC 3 x LUNGES

The important thing is to try all of the Strength MOVEs and learn how each one benefits the body differently. Once you are familiar with all the exercises, pick the ones that address your need in the moment.

Look back to your Moving towards Goals sheet and see if you had a goal to increase strength and muscle tone. Connect this goal to the MOVEs you will do this week and use either the ThinkMOVE App or the daily journal to track your moves and reflect on your experience of doing strength MOVE breaks.

Try doing the strength exercises three times a day every day this week, and take note of the effects they have in the middle of your day.

When you practice strength moves, try to remember to breathe consciously and be aware of your body's position (REMEMBER: healthy positions: FASH).

TEAM MOVE CHALLENGE: In your teams or with a colleague/ friend, challenge each other each day to do as many strength MOVEs as possible. You can create competitions for each day and for the whole week. For example, who can do the most number of SQUATS/PUSH UPS/ DEADLIFTS per day.

Finally, plan and strategize together any barriers (e.g., travel, work-load) that may get in the way of you doing MOVE breaks this week.

14. Week Five: Cardio and Stringing

Objectives for Week Five: Cardio and Stringing

- Learn about the benefits of cardio MOVEs and overcome the stigma of moving at work.
- Learn a series of cardio moves and increase energy throughout the day naturally.
- Use stress (feeling trigger) as a way to trigger MOVE breaks and cope with stress in a healthy way.
- For the team to have fun moving together try cardio MOVEs and encourage a culture of healthy movement at the office.

14.1 Week five lesson

This week we are focusing on cardio MOVEs, which will bring ener-gy and fun into your day at the office. We've saved cardio MOVEs for one of the last weeks of the introductory program because they really break through the chains of the sedentary culture.

Out of all the MOVES, cardio is one of the best ways to generate energy because it stimulates the entire body and increases blood flow.

Movement generates energy. Also, cardio MOVEs are a great way to physically embody the act of moving past psychological stuck points. There may be times in your day where you feel stuck or overwhelmed. Taking 30–60 seconds to do a cardio MOVE can create a mindset shift because you are deciding to get up, do something good for your body, and shake off stress and tension.

Hopefully by now, you have created some strong movement roots with various triggers and movements so that you are now ready to add cardio MOVEs.

Benefits of cardio moves:

- **Increase energy:** Get your whole body moving and feel the boost of energy that can be a healthy replacement for that second cup of coffee you typically reach for at 3:00 p.m.

- **Exercise, particularly cardiovascular exercise improves the brain's functioning:** Research is showing that higher cognitive processes called executive functions are improved by bouts of cardio exercise. These include abilities like sustaining attention, regulating emotions, shifting attention, planning, and memory.

- **Gain focus and creativity:** By increasing blood flow to the prefrontal cortex, your ability to focus, learn, and problem solve creatively will increase.

- **Improve heart health:** Incorporating short bouts of cardio MOVEs can be an efficient way of getting in exercise that stimulates the cardiovascular system and helps improve and maintain a healthy heart for many years to come.

- **Increase your metabolism:** Research demonstrates improvements in insulin sensitivity and lowered glucose levels through short intermittent bouts of high intensity, cardio-based exercise.

- **Helps with weight loss:** Cardio exercise is an important component of any healthy weight loss program and in the maintenance of a healthy weight. Our bodies were designed for movement so even something as simple as going for a walk for 20 to 60 minutes can provide most of the benefits of any exercise program including reaching or maintaining a healthy weight.

- **Stimulates the musculoskeletal and digestive system:** Cardio MOVEs like jogging on the spot or invisible jump rope will stimulate your muscles and bones by the increased gravitational pull. This will prevent muscle and bone atrophy. Also moving around will help keep things moving in terms of digestion, and improve gut health.

- **Shakes off the stress:** ThinkMOVE is all about breaking patterns. When we are stressed out and stuck in the seated position, stress can pile on us. Getting up and doing something cardio-based is a way of shaking off that stress and connecting to something that's more important than any momentary stress: our health. Our bodies can help anchor us and we will be more capable of facing the challenges and stresses of the day.

- **Reduces risk for chronic illness like heart disease, diabetes, and cancer**: Clearly, by improving the health indicators discussed above, we will also reduce the risk of developing chronic and preventable illnesses.

14.2 Week five exercise: Cardio

See Figures 42 to 45.

14.3 Week five practice

Continue to use the triggers from the previous weeks and add one stress-based trigger.

Think about situations that cause you stress regularly throughout your work day. Perhaps you can recall something from week one when you practiced the body awareness exercises.

Pick one specific stress trigger so that whenever you feel it, you'll use it as a signal to take a MOVE break. An example might be, "When I notice myself stressed about the amount of email I have, I will take a minute to MOVE and ground myself again."

Try to aim for seven or eight MOVE breaks per day (MPD); also, try to do three cardio MOVEs every day or pick a goal that is challenging and realistic for you. Focus the rest of your MOVEs on body awareness and flexibility, leaving balance and strength MOVEs for now.

There are four different cardio exercises. Try all four of them and see which ones you like the most. Going for a walk or having walking meetings also count as cardio MOVEs, so if you do take a walk remember to input these into the ThinkMOVE app and get credit for your MOVES!

Consult your Moving towards Goals sheet and see if you had a goal to increase energy, manage stress better, or lose weight. Connect this goal to the cardio MOVEs you will do this week and record your experiences and reflections of the cardio MOVE breaks. Whether you write/type it or not, do take a brief moment to ask yourself how it felt to do a cardio MOVE and anchor any positive effects you notice so that you will be encouraged to practice it again in the future.

Try cardio MOVEs three times a day this week. Try doing these cardio MOVEs with a partner or your whole team to help overcome the barriers to moving at the office. Try scheduling in one cardio MOVE every day with your team so you can practice with some social support.

Desk Jogging

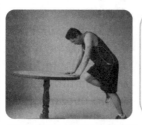

1. Place your hands on your desk and your body in a plank position.
2. Begin jogging on the spot.
3. Do mini push ups as you go!
4. Imagine you are on a stationary bike!
5. Try alternating between fast and slow. Have fun!

Muscles used: Whole body, legs.
Benefits: Engages upper and lower body; stimulates the heart and aerobic capacity.
Aim for: Do 60 seconds; you can vary intensity/speed throughout.
Modifications: Bring the knees up higher to increase intensity.
Watch out for: <u>Starting off too fast;</u> take your time warming up, try going faster at the end.

Figure 42

Invisible Jump Rope or Jumping

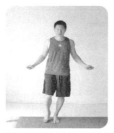

1. Imagine jumping rope with your hands swinging the rope by your side.
2. You can jump up and down, side to side, on one foot, then the next. Maybe even a double-jump or two?

Muscles used: Entire body, particularly legs and shoulders.
Benefits: Great cardio workout, G-forces from jumping prevent bone density loss and muscle atrophy.
Aim for: One to two minutes.
Modifications: If jumping is too hard on your knees, try bouncing without leaving the floor.
Watch out for: Make sure your body is in a good position and your abs are engaged.

Figure 43

Jogging on the Spot

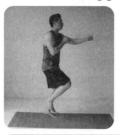

1. Start jogging on the spot.
2. Add punches.
3. To vary the intensity, increase the speed of the jog and punches, and bring knees up higher.

Muscles used: Whole body.
Benefits: Great cardio move that engages both upper and lower body. Can vary intensity easily.
Aim for: One to two minutes.
Modifications: You can throw jabs and uppercuts; you can run faster on the spot.
Watch out for: Hitting other people! Be mindful of your space.

Figure 44

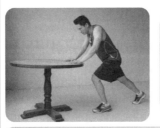

Desk Mountain Climbing

1. Start with hands on the desk and legs in lunges position.
2. Hop on your legs so the forward leg goes back and the back leg forward.
3. Continue for one minute.

Muscles used: Whole body.
Benefits: Excellent cardio move with explosive jumps to get the heart pumping!
Aim for: One to two minutes.
Modifications: Change your pace to increase/decrease intensity; widen or shorten stance.
Watch out for: Holding your breath; going too quickly. *Always start slowly.*

Figure 45

When you practice cardio MOVEs, ensure that your wardrobe is safe to do the move. If you're wearing high heels for example, it would be a good idea to kick them off for the minute it will take to the MOVE break.

TEAM MOVE: In your teams or with a colleague/trusted friend, share what your stress-based trigger is for this week. Discuss why you picked this trigger and what you hope to experience doing a MOVE break in response to it.

Finally, plan and strategize together how to remove any barriers (e.g., travel, workload) that may get in the way of you doing MOVE breaks this week.

15. Week Six: Whole Body Integration

Objectives for week six: Whole body integration

- Review all triggers and select the top three triggers that worked well for you.

- Mix different MOVE categories together to create powerful MOVE breaks combinations.

- Personalize your MOVEs to your body and goals.

- Increase your total MOVE per days (MPDs) to eight to ten a day.

- Reflect on all that you have learned and changed in the past six weeks and celebrate with your team.

15.1 Week six lesson

Congratulations, you made it to the last week of the six-week introductory ThinkMOVE program.

This week, we will be reviewing all that you have learned and helping you create an individualized ThinkMOVE plan. You'll reflect on what your specific goals are now that you have completed the six weeks and how best to continue practicing movement throughout your day.

In this final week, we are going to learn how to combine the five MOVE categories of body awareness, flexibility, balance, strength, and cardio into individual MOVE breaks so you can begin to increase the effectiveness of each by incorporating the benefits from the categories.

If you have been doing one-minute MOVE breaks, perhaps now is the time to extend them to two minutes.

Before we get to goal-setting and creating your unique ThinkMOVE program, let's review the various triggers you have learned.

In week one you practiced scheduling three MOVE breaks into your day. You scheduled some individually and some with your team. Scheduling is really powerful because it roots movement into your day and becomes the starting point for stringing many moves together.

In week two, you practiced feeling/physical sensation-based triggers. These might have been feelings of soreness, tiredness, or worry. These are powerful triggers because they are the signals that let you know what's going on within your body and the needs that are asking for your attention. They enable you to address small issues before they become larger health issues.

In week three, you learned to use behavioral triggers. For example, going to the washroom or checking social media were easy-to-identify moments when a MOVE break might be needed. A natural movement that stems from a behavioral trigger might be choosing to take the stairs over the elevator.

In week four, you used social or environmental triggers. For example, instead of using the phone or email, actually walking over and talking to your colleague face-to-face and inviting him or her to MOVE with you. This might look as simple as standing up, perhaps stretching, or even going for a walking meeting.

In week five, you used stress as a feeling-based trigger. You identified particular situations or moments in your day where you felt consistently stressed or overwhelmed and used this as a cue to do a MOVE. This was also the week where you learned to do cardio MOVEs at work, which hopefully helped you shake off the stress.

Throughout the program, you have been using the ThinkMOVE app as a tool for triggering MOVES, referencing exercises, and tracking your total MOVE breaks. You might also be using a wearable technology like a Fitbit or a pedometer. These are all great ways of initiating and tracking your movement.

You can think of these various triggers as a web: The more triggers you use, the greater your network, the stronger your ability to disrupt sedentary time.

Look back. Which were the top three triggers for you? Look at Figure 46 for a refresher and then fill out Exercise 13.

INTERNAL TRIGGERS	EXTERNAL TRIGGERS
• FEELINGS	• TIME (SCHEDULING)
• PHYSICAL SENSATIONS	• ENVIRONMENTAL
• THOUGHTS	• SOCIAL
• BEHAVIOR	• TOOLS (APPS)

Figure 46

Exercise 13
Top Three Triggers for Movement

My top three triggers for MOVEMENT are:

_____
_____
_____

Additional ways/contexts to practice my favorite triggers:

_____
_____
_____

15.1a The psychological and social benefits of each of the five categories of MOVE

We will review each of the categories so that you can make decisions about which categories are a priority for you as you design your Think-MOVE program. Now that you've had a chance to learn and practice each of the MOVEs from the various categories, you have a better understanding of how each category can be used.

Body awareness is foundational to listening and understanding the body's needs. This includes listening to specific elements of the body such as breathing, body position, and tensions. The act of listening to your body helps put you in connection to yourself so that you can feel better and work better.

As you have been learning to move throughout your day, all of the exercises you have learned are unique opportunities to listen and learn about the positive impacts movement can have on your body and your health. For example, what do flexibility MOVEs do for you that is different from strength MOVEs?

Flexibility MOVEs are great for increasing mobility and range of motion. Psychologically, they are a great way of letting go of tensions being held in the body and practicing going with the flow.

Balance MOVEs are a way to practice being present, centered, and self-aware. These are opportunities to experience your efforts in the face of challenge. At the same time as exerting effort, there is a lightness to balance MOVEs that encourage us to not take ourselves too seriously. Finding the balance (pun intended!) between effort and effortlessness is the key to balance MOVEs.

Strength MOVEs are a way of creating structure and building inner and outer strength. A strength challenge in the middle of your day, perhaps with squats or push ups, gives you a clear and concrete task that you can face and overcome. This can provide an experience of confidence, which can be very helpful in the face of an otherwise chaotic day.

Cardio MOVEs are the most challenging in terms of overcoming the sedentary culture. These MOVEs are an opportunity to practice caring about yourself and your health and not the opinions or judgments of other people. The ideal situation would be if the team could support one another and move together to do these active and engaging moves.

15.2 Week six exercise: Combining what you've learned

Instead of learning new MOVEs, this week practice mixing and combining each of the five categories into unique pairings. Here are four combos I think you'll love:

> Option 1. Flexibility with strength. Starting off with a flexibility MOVE will help you shake off the tension accumulated

from a period of sitting and prepare the body for a more active MOVE such as strength. A great pairing would be mountain bends with squats. You can either do 30/30 seconds for a one-minute MOVE break or 60/60 for a two-minute break.

Option 2. Strength with cardio. This is a higher intensity MOVE break and will really get your heart pumping. The idea is to warm up, perhaps doing some light desk push ups for 30 to 60 seconds, and then you might transition to desk jogging for another 30 to 60 seconds to kick it up a notch.

Option 3. Flexibility with balance. The flexibility MOVE will help loosen and free the body of the stiffness of being in a chair. When you try the balance MOVE, you will be more in tune with your body so you can bring greater presence and focus to the movement.

Option 4. Flexibility with cardio. Starting with a stretch is a great way to get the body in gear to do a more intense cardio MOVE. You can think of the first MOVE as an appetizer to warm up your belly and the second MOVE as the main course. In this sense, when you are tracking your MOVE breaks with the ThinkMOVE journal you might select your focal point as the second MOVE so that you can track what MOVEs you are doing.

15.3 Week six practice

Revisit your Moving towards Goals worksheet. Review what you wrote six weeks ago and reflect on what you have achieved and experienced from the program. What health goals remain and what new goals would you like to pursue?

Here is a stem to help you write out your vision: "Seeing and experiencing myself reaching my ideal health a year from now, I am experiencing … " (Consider your feelings, relationships, and your work. Also, what changes would people notice about you from the outside?)

Try to aim for eight to ten MOVE breaks per day (MPDs) or pick a goal that is challenging and realistic for you.

Try to do two MOVE combos every day. You could do these based on the program that you've created for yourself or you can select two MOVE categories that you would like to combine based on your needs.

TEAM MOVE: In your teams or with a colleague/trusted friend, share what your top three triggers are from the program. Discuss why you picked these triggers and how exactly you plan on practicing these triggers in your day.

Also, share your goals and plans for yourself in the ThinkMOVE program. See if you can enlist others who share the same goal as you to join the program with you.

Finally, plan and strategize overcoming any barriers (e.g., travel, workload) that may get in the way of you doing MOVE breaks this week.

Exercise 14
Specific Goals

Here is a list of some specific health areas. In addition to checking the boxes that apply, write out **specific details** below. Wherever possible be clear and specific about how these changes will be **observed** or **measured**.

☐ What changes would you notice in terms of your **energy**? For example, an increase in energy, mental clarity (initiative, focus, productivity, etc.).

I will notice my energy _____

☐ Weight loss — e.g., I will lose 15 pounds, feel more confident

I will lose _____ lbs and feel _____

☐ What differences would you notice in how you **feel**? For example, better mood, feel happier, more positive outlook

I will feel _____

☐ What changes would you notice in **your coworkers/team**? For example, better team connection or a happier team

With my colleagues I will notice _____

☐ Pain: less stiffness, soreness, numbness and pain: more flexibility, mobility, and ease (for example, neck, back, shoulders, legs)

In my body I will notice _____

☐ Increased job satisfaction:

I will feel _____

☐ Improved strength:

I will be able to_____

☐ Improved cardio:

I will be able to _____

☐ Improved flexibility:

I will be able to _____

☐ Improved body awareness: awareness, posture, breathing:

I will notice _____

☐ Improved self-confidence or sense of attractiveness:

  I will see myself as

☐ Improved balance/coordination:

  I will be able to _____

☐ Increased muscle tone:

  I will notice _____

☐ Improved appearance:

  I will look _____

☐ Improved stress management:

  I will be able to _____

Now based on your reflection of your goals, how would you allocate ten MOVE breaks into the five categories? (*Imagine you have 10 Poker Chips to distribute to each category*)

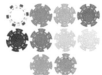

Body Awareness	Flexibility	Balance	Strength	Cardio

To create an overall program that is balanced and personalized, you would allocate two MOVE chips into each of the five categories. Then each day you would aim to do one of each MOVE type perhaps starting with Body Awareness, then Flexibility and doing one of each until you reached Cardio. That would be five MOVE breaks. Then you would repeat the cycle starting with Body Awareness again.

If you have allocated three or more MOVE breaks to any category, that's probably because you have a focused goal that you are trying to achieve and it's a priority for you.

For example, a person who wants to increase strength and improve energy might use the following program:

Body Awareness	Flexibility	Balance	Strength	Cardio
2	2	0	3	3

Below is a plan for each day of the MOVE type and number of MOVE breaks.

MONDAY	TUESDAY	WEDNESDAY	THURSDAY	FRIDAY
BODY AWARE	BODY AWARE	BODY AWARE	BODY AWARE	BODY AWARE
2	2	2	2	2
FLEXIBILITY	FLEXIBILITY	FLEXIBILITY	FLEXIBILITY	FLEXIBILITY
2	2	2	2	2
STRENGTH	*CARDIO*	*STRENGTH*	*CARDIO*	*STRENGTH*
3	3	3	3	3

For more specific goals, such as weight loss or energy boosting, we provide specific programs that will help you with those specific goals. You can graduate to these after completing the six-week program as described in Chapter 6.

7
Health Defined

Definitions of health vary greatly from one person to the next. Some people think of health as primarily a physical ideal, like having chiseled abs, or being athletic or strong. For others, health relates more to a state of mind, which ideally might be energized, happy, and productive. For a great majority however, health is not something they have clearly defined, or isn't something that enters their conscious awareness until a problem occurs like an injury, significant weight gain, or illness. Given the demands and the blur of daily living, health often takes a back seat and that is unfortunate since health is the fuel that allows us to create, connect, and fulfill our potential.

It is helpful to define health not only negatively (i.e., the absence of problems) but to also create a positive definition and vision of health so the goals at which we are aiming are clear, measurable, and achievable. Having a positive definition of health can empower us to go beyond mere survival and enter a state of thriving that enables us to grow.

Health is the total renewable resources, which includes energy, ability and time you have available to do what you want and need in life that is unhindered by limitations, physical, mental and social, such as illness, injury, fatigue, or toxic relationships.

In this definition, health is not an all or nothing state. Rather, it is a resource that fluctuates moment by moment (at a moment in time) depending on how you are using your body, the amount of exercise you do, what foods you consume, your environment, the amount of sleep you get, the stress and demands in your life, and your relationships. Health can be assessed based on how much health resource (energy, ability, and time) you have available to you.

To be clear, health is a limited resource because no one gets out of this life alive. However, to a certain extent, health resources are renewable. We can renew certain aspects of our body and slow the deterioration of health and the aging process with consistent healing practices. Strength training, for example, helps regenerate the body with new and larger muscle tissues. As well, aerobic exercise has been shown to increase neurogenesis and neuroplasticity: the production of new neurons (brain cells) and new connections between neurons. The ThinkMOVE program incorporates strength and aerobic training for these reasons. We'll review the healing side of health in greater depth later.

As discussed in previous chapters, prolonged sitting accelerates the aging process while movement heals. In the ThinkMOVE program, regular and short movement breaks are used to help heal the body from the costly effects of being sedentary. Moving frequently throughout the day offsets the cost of prolonged sitting by keeping the body healthy and stimulating hormonal, digestive, and musculoskeletal systems, which require movement to be activated.

Health resources refer to three major elements: energy, ability, and time. Energy is the capacity of the mind and body to do sustained work and is an essential component of health resource. During the goal setting phase, more than 90 percent of the participants in the ThinkMOVE program said that they would like more energy. For some, more energy meant being able to sustain focus and attention for longer periods of time at work. For others, it meant having more mental and physical energy to help the kids with their homework or to play with them after a long day at work.

Another component of health resource is the ability of your mind and body to do the things we want and need to do. For example, the physical ability to carry groceries, take the stairs, to walk and play sports, or the mental ability to focus, remember information, or problem solve. With the ThinkMOVE program, mental and physical abilities are enhanced by improving body awareness, flexibility, strength, balance, and cardio.

Time is a difficult element of health resource to discuss since no one can predict how much time they have left to live. However, it is clear the amount of time we have to live is an important resource and is directly tied to the state of our health. The best we can do is learn from health science and population studies to predict which behaviors could result in the longest, healthiest life possible. In 2009, the average life expectancy in Canada was 80 years for men and 84 years for women. But our health resource is not just the total amount of time we have on this planet, but time in combination with one's energies and abilities all contribute to a person's quality of life.

1. Health Spending

Just like any resource, like money, health can be spent and it can be earned. These are the two sides of the health equation. We spend our health on things like a day of work, taking care of the family, and doing chores. There are four major ways you can spend health. These categories are not mutually exclusive and may overlap. They are:

1. Stress spending

2. Indulgent spending

3. Practical spending

4. Flow spending

Stress spending represents the least productive type of spending. It occurs when we are spinning our wheels and our energy is being spent with no clear benefit or action. Some degree of stress is normal and expected in the face of the demands of daily living. Stress goes up significantly during a major life change or transition. However, when stress spending reaches high levels and stays there, it creates an unsustainable pattern of being overwhelmed and eventual burnout.

An example might be an employee, let's call him Ken, who is having insecure thoughts about his abilities or a low sense of his worth. These insecurities could result from a situation where Ken is feeling undervalued by management and is having anxieties that he will be passed over for a promotion, or even laid off. Depending on the work culture and the quality of communication between Ken and his manager, and Ken's capacity and willingness to bring up concerns, things may be left unspoken. Ken may get caught up in overwhelming stress and anxiety which he keeps to himself. With no resolution in sight, Ken engages in ruminative thinking where there is little to no return or reward, just cost to his health resources. In this example, Ken is spending his health resources (time, energy, and ability) on his imagined fears about the future (being laid off or missing out on promotional opportunities), feelings of resentment against his employer, and/or low feelings about his self worth. Although there is little to no benefit in getting caught in stress spending of this kind, it isn't easy to get unstuck from these patterns; at least not without support and understanding from friends, colleagues, family, and sometimes professional supports.

However a person experiences stress, these experiences undoubtedly have a significant cost to health. Early experiences of stress spending may be feeling overwhelmed and worried which may later manifest as depression or anxiety. These conditions can eventually escalate to a state of burnout where one's health resources are emptied and the individual is paralyzed to act. Burnout is a situation where an individual's challenges, problems, and work demands outweigh and overwhelm his or her ability, resources, and skill to cope. This is an extremely unsustainable state and can result in serious health consequences such as mental illness, nervous breakdown, high blood pressure, ulcers, cancer, and heart attacks. Overwhelming stress can be seen as a signal that an individual's capacity and skill with coping with the demands of his or her life may need support and/or growth. Improving one's coping abilities could involve processing one's emotional experience and expanding one's perspective and abilities to cope in therapy or coaching. It could also occur relationally by learning skills to have open and direct communication within an organization.

Becoming aware of your stress spending gives you some choices that might not have been visible to you previously. Stress can be reduced and even transformed with a change in perspective, mindset, and attitude. Stress can also be reduced by having a clear plan and receiving support to put it into action.

Indulgent spending is done on activities that are meant to be pleasurable, like taking a week's vacation at a beachfront resort or, on a smaller scale, eating a box of chocolates. Indulging the sense with inspiring music, breathtaking views, aromatic smells, sensual touches, and savory foods is part of the joy of living. It can be a welcome relief from the daily demands of work and practical matters.

Indulgent spending has a complex role to play when it comes to health. It is the source of pleasure but it also a way to take a break from the discipline of healthy behaviors like exercise and healthy eating. For some, moments of indulgent spending help refuel willpower, but for others it is a slippery slope to be avoided.

Sometimes indulgent spending can result in pain when done in excess and without conscious awareness. A daily habit of sitting in front of the TV eating chips is an example of indulgent spending that has a costly price to health for temporary pleasure. The specific costs include weight gain, muscle atrophy, and increased risk for heart disease and cancer. For some, the pleasure is worth the cost and for others it is not. This a personal decision and no one has the right to determine what is correct for another person. What's useful is making conscious choices about how much indulgent spending to engage in as it relates to one's ideal vision of health.

Practical spending involves using one's health resources to do the things that need to get done to maintain basic levels of functioning. For example, using your energy to go to the dentist, to clean, do laundry, pay bills, and do paperwork: These practical items need to get done in order for life to function smoothly. They require little skill and effort except perhaps in getting started. For some people, these things tend to feel boring and mundane. Sometimes when these practical demands are neglected they become a looming burden which contributes to stress spending. So pay that bill that's been sitting on your desk, already!

Sometimes what you spend on your health actually energizes you and adds to your health and vitality. When we are engaged in our passion and mission in life this is called flow spending. The word "flow" is inspired by the psychologist Mihaly Csìkszentmihályi's work on flow. Flow is the state of consciousness where someone is so absorbed in an activity that they experience:

1. Intense and focused concentration on the present moment

2. Merging of action and awareness

3. A loss of self-consciousness

4. A sense of personal control or agency over the situation or activity

5. A distortion of time; one's subjective experience of time is altered, either slowed or sped up

6. Experience of the activity as intrinsically rewarding (positive emotions)

Some examples of flow spending might be working on an exciting project or creative work about which you are passionate and that you find fulfilling and meaningful. When you have found work that energizes you and gives you a feeling of vitality and focus, you know you've created a situation sustainable for your health. The scope of flow spending could be as small as trying a painting class or as large as inventing an environmentally friendly car. In some situations, practical spending and flow spending can be experienced simultaneously. For example, a parent helping his son with his math homework and finding that perfect way to explain a concept that helps his son understand.

When you spend your health resources on creating the experiences that truly matter to you, health and vitality increase. Asking questions like, "How are you spending your health?," "Are my skills and abilities being challenged?," "Are there times when I am so engaged in an activity that I lose a sense of time and self-consciousness?," and "Do my activities feel significant and meaningful?" are ways of clarifying whether you have opportunities to engage in flow spending.

Figure 47 is a chart that organizes the four types of health resource spending with examples. They vary according to the amount of reward experienced and the effort and skill required.

	High Reward	Low Reward
High Effort/Skill	**FLOW** **(Playing piano)**	**STRESS** **(Worrying)**
Low Effort/Skill	**PRACTICAL** **(Washing dishes)**	**INDULGENT** **(Eating a box of chocolate)**

Figure 47

After a day of exertion, our bodies need adequate rest so that they can heal, cells and tissues can regenerate, and we can do it all over again the next day. This is the way we earn our health. In this next section we will explore the ways we earn back our health with the idea that there is a healing side to health.

2. The Healing Side of Health

Have you ever noticed the word "heal" within the word "health"? For optimal health to exist, there needs to be a consistent practice of healing the body from the natural wear and tear of daily living. This should include healing both the body and the mind. Your health needs proper care and regular maintenance just like a car, yet few people give themselves the time and attention their body deserves. Healing is the collection of behaviors, strategies, and habits that help the body recover and regenerate after exertion. Some examples of things that help the body and mind heal include regular movement, sleep, meditation, water, walks outside, time with friends, massage therapy, psychotherapy, music, exercise, art, naps, nutrient-rich foods, vacation, journaling, or spiritual practices.

The importance of balancing spending with healing can be seen within the very structure of our nervous system. The nervous system is divided into two main branches: the sympathetic nervous system which helps put our body into action, and the parasympathetic system which helps us relax and recover. The activity of the sympathetic nervous system can be seen as the system that helps us spend our health on the experiences that matter and the function of the parasympathetic can be seen as the system that aids in our efforts to heal and recover our health.

Many people are unaware of the relationship between the healing and spending sides of health often resulting in neglecting any healing practices in their lives. They work long hours, take on more projects, skip meals, lose sleep and indulge in cigarettes, drugs, and alcohol to stay afloat. This is like living life on credit cards without a source of income to pay off the accumulating debt.

Optimizing health resources requires attention to spending as well as practices of healing which replenish and regenerate the total health resources available. The workaholic tendency in our culture tends to result in the neglect of the healing side of health. Some work cultures perceive healing practices as unnecessary, a waste of time, or even a sign of weakness. However, just as breathing works better when you combine inhaling with exhaling, health resources can be optimized and made sustainable when spending is balanced with healing.

The healing side of health can be divided into two paths: passive and active. Passive forms of healing are periods of minimal activity which allow for recovery and regeneration of the body and mental energy. Active healing requires more effort and often involves movement. They also aid in recovery, but they primarily help elevate one's physical and mental energy capacity to new limits so you can do more for longer.

See Figure 48.

Time alone is an abstraction that is easily taken for granted. Being aware of the choices you make as they relate to the cost and benefits to your health resources empowers you to make better and more conscious decisions about your health resources.

Being sedentary has clear costs to health. As this book has hopefully demonstrated, we can do many things to offset the impact of this behavior by simply disrupting prolonged sitting with periodic bouts of movement.

Active Healing	Passive Healing
• Exercise (strength, aerobic) • Stretch (dynamic/static, e.g., yoga) • MOVE every 20 to 40 minutes • Journal (reflect on the day and the future) • Foam rolling • Connect with friends, family • Appreciate and be grateful • Go for a walk • Find solitude	• Sleep • Eat nutrient-rich foods • Drink water • Breathe deep • Nap • Take mental breaks • Meditate • Listen to music

Figure 48

Exercise 15
Two Questions

Try getting into the habit of asking yourself many times throughout the day:

"How am I spending my health right now?"

Assess whether the activity is worthy of your energy, abilities, and time.

When you can answer this question congruently and feel satisfied that you are spending your health on things that truly matter, you will inevitably feel more alive, energetic, and vital.

Also, try to get into the habit of asking yourself throughout the day:

"How am I healing my health today?"

Creating habits and rituals of healing will ensure that you are able to perform optimally in all areas of your life since you will have the energy, ability, and time to do what you want and need.

3. Optimizing Health: Spend Wisely, Heal Frequently

In order to optimize health, individuals can begin to practice spending health resources wisely and healing them frequently. There is no one-size-fits-all formula for this. People will vary according to which areas of spending they value most and which healing practices fit with their personality and lifestyle. Every person is capable of making conscious choices that optimize the spending and healing sides of health that fit their unique lifestyle and values.

Spending wisely means making conscious choices about how you use your health resources. "Healing frequently" is a gentle encouragement to take care of those health resources through proper maintenance and recovery practices for the body.

It is never enough to know what to do. You also need the knowledge and skill to do it. This is particularly true when it comes to creating healthy habits. Many people start off with the best of intentions, but then get lost in myriad details and fads.

The details of how to do the program from here on out are individually determined. The lists below are merely suggestions that can be used as a guide. Your efforts, exploration and experimentation will help you design your own practices and habits.

Here is a list of possible activities and guidelines from which to choose in Figure 49.

Spend Wisely	Heal Frequently
• Make conscious choices about how you use health resources (energy, abilities, and time) • Spend resources in a way that balances your needs as well as significant others'. • Engage in pursuits that are meaningful and significant (i.e., flow spending) to you. • Express your creativity whether that is in music, visual arts, writing, technology, or design. • Be aware of stress spending and make efforts to resolve or heal these patterns by receiving support and help from colleagues, friends, family, or professionals. • Indulge consciously and moderately. • Don't lose sight of important areas of practical spending.	• Take regular MOVE breaks, one every 20-40 minutes of prolonged sitting. • Eat healthy, nutrient-rich meals. • Get adequate amounts of sleep every night. • Practice deep breathing. • Appreciate what you have; practice gratitude. • Drink water. • Connect with friends regularly. • Stretch regularly. • Spend quality time with family. • Take time to relax and savor the present moment. • Celebrate accomplishments, milestones, and life itself!

Figure 49

So far we have talked about health as a resource similar to money. Although there are similarities, it's important to see health as a separate and distinct resource that has a unique value. Often, businesses want to know how a program like ThinkMOVE will contribute to the financial bottom line. Research demonstrates the return on investment ranges from $1.50 to $6.15 for every dollar spent on health and wellness. But what good is money if you have no energy? If you lose the ability to move or run out of time due to premature death? No doubt money is important. It makes the world go round, but money can't be enjoyed without a healthy hand to receive and spend it. This is why I believe that health is a more valuable resource than money and therefore we should prioritize our health over money.

8
Health Resource
Self-Assessment (HRSA)

The Health Resource Self-Assessment (HRSA) is a self-assessment tool that helps you determine your level of health resources, specifically the patterns of your health spending in comparison to your healing practices. In this book you have been introduced to a method of taking care of your health that addresses sitting time. Now is a good time to reflect on your experience of health: how you are spending it and how you are healing it. The HRSA can be done at any time, but it may be particularly useful as you begin to engage the practice of moving throughout the day. Getting a baseline measure of how you spend and heal can motivate you to use your health wisely.

Consider each of the four health spending types described in Chapter 7 (flow, practical, indulgent, and stress) and create a score out of 10 which represents how much energy you spend on each dimension. For flow spending, 10 represents you spend the most energy you could ever possibly hope to spend on flow; a 0 represents that you don't spend any energy doing things that are flow-related.

For healing practices you will create a score out of 20 for each of the two healing types (passive and active).

You will create two scores out of 40 for spending and for healing and subtract spending from healing to determine your overall health resource score. At the end of the assessment you will see some information which will explain the meaning of your score.

Exercise 16
Health Resource Spending Assessment (HRSA)

Consider how often or how true each item is for you and how much you use your health resources for each type of health spending:

0: never/not at all true;

1: rarely/moderately true;

2: very true/most of the time/as much as I would like

Some items are more weighted than others. Multiply these items by two ("X 2") and add all the numbers in each section to create a score out of 20. For the four categories of spending you will divide your score out of 20 by two to create a spending score out of 40.

HEALTH RESOURCE SELF-ASSESSMENT (HRSA)

Spending Type	Items	Rating Score
FLOW	☐ Do you enjoy your work and find it rewarding?	___/2 **X2**
	☐ Are you engaged in creating things or experiences that interest you and your value?	___/2
	☐ Do you find your work/effort/activities meaningful, significant?	___/2
	☐ Do your efforts have a positive impact on the world?	___/2
	☐ Do you feel the challenges you face match your skill level?	___/2
	☐ Are you ever so engaged and focused in your work that you lose a sense of time? A loss of self-consciousness?	___/2
	☐ Do you experience activities that are intrinsically rewarding (doing them is a reward in itself)?	___/2 **X2**
	☐ Do you have opportunities to collaborate with others in a way that is rewarding, energizing, or fun?	___/2
FLOW SCORE (TOTAL OUT OF 20 ÷ 2)		**___/10**
PRACTICAL	☐ Do you pay your bills on time?	___/2
	☐ Do you spend enough time cleaning and organizing your space at home or work?	___/2
	☐ Do you keep a tidy and organized desk?	___/2
	☐ Do you spend time meeting family?	___/2
	☐ Do you get to projects around the house?	___/2
	☐ Do you properly maintain your car?	___/2
	☐ Do you complete or address practical matters in your life?	___/2 **X2**
	☐ When it comes to practical tasks, do you avoid procrastination?	___/2 **X2**
PRACTICAL SCORE (TOTAL OUT OF 20 ÷ 2)		**___/10**

INDULGENT	How often are you on social media?	__/2
	How frequently do you watch TV/Netflix?	__/2
	How often do you eat junk food/sweets?	__/2
	How often do you eat out?	__/2
	How often do you have sex?	__/2
	How often do you use drugs/alcohol?	__/2
	How often do you take vacation/travel?	__/2
	How often do you sleep in?	__/2
	How often would you say you experience indulgent pleasure in your life?	__/2 **X2**
INDULGENT SCORE (TOTAL OUT OF 20 ÷ 2)		**__/10**
STRESS	How much anxiety/worry do you experience?	__/2
	How much depression do you experience?	__/2
	How true is this statement: I do not feel in control of what happens in my life.	__/2 **X2**
	How much irritability or impatience do you experience?	__/2
	How often do you check email?	__/2
	How often do you ruminate about problems at work/home?	__/2
	How much stress do you currently experience at home and work?	__/2 **X2**
	How likely are you to try solve problems on your own rather than ask for help?	__/2
STRESS SCORE (TOTAL OUT OF 20 ÷ 2)		**__/10**

Healing Practice

Consider how often or how true each item is for you and how much you engage in these health healing behaviors/practices.

   0 = never/not at all true;

   1 = rarely/moderately true;

   2 = most of the time/very true/ as much as I would like)

Some items are weighted more than others. Multiply these items by two (as indicated) and in each section create a score out of 20.

Type of healing	Items	Rating Score
ACTIVE HEALING	How often do you exercise (strength, aerobic)?	__/2
	How often do you stretch/loosen the body (dynamic/static/yoga)?	__/2
	Do you MOVE every 20 to 40 minutes?	__/2 **X2**
	Do you journal or spend time reflecting on the day that has occurred and the future?	__/2
	Do you get massages regularly?	__/2
	Do you practice appreciation or gratitude?	__/2
	How often do you connect with friends and family?	__/2
	How often do you engage in practices that help your body recover and regain energy?	__/2 **X2**
ACTIVE HEALING SCORE (TOTAL OUT OF 20 POINTS)		**__/20**

ACTIVE HEALING SCORE (TOTAL OUT OF 20 POINTS)		____/20
PASSIVE HEALING	☐ Do you get enough sleep?	___/2 **X2**
	☐ Do you eat regular and healthy meals?	___/2 **X2**
	☐ Do you drink enough water every day?	___/2
	☐ Do you take vitamins/supplements or ensure that you get the vitamins and minerals you need from whole foods?	___/2
	☐ Do you engage in meditation/relaxation/spiritual practices that help re-energize you?	___/2
	☐ Do you take naps?	___/2
	☐ Do you take regular mental breaks away from screens and other stimuli?	___/2 **X2**
PASSIVE HEALING SCORE (TOTAL OUT OF 20 POINTS)		____/20
TOTAL HEALING SCORE out of 20 X 2		____/40

HEALTH SCORE = SPENDING – HEALING

Here is an example:

Flow	6 /10	Active healing	10/20
Practical	7 /10		
Indulgent	8 /10	Passive healing	14/20
Stress	8 /10		
Total spending	**29** /40	**Total healing**	**24/40**

In this example (29-24) this individual would receive a score of +5.

Input your scores here:

Flow	___/10	Active healing	___/20
Practical	___/10		
Indulgent	___/10	Passive healing	___/20
Stress	___/10		
Total spending	___ /40	**Total healing**	___/40

Total Spending (_____) – Total Healing (_____) = _____

(0 > ...) Health Resource Rich: Any negative number means you have more health resources than you are currently spending. Lucky you!

(0-10) Health Resource Optimizing: You are likely feeling that you are in a healthy well balanced place and that you have enough energy to meet the demands of your life.

(10-20) Health Resource Overspending: You are likely experiencing a great deal of stress and a feeling that you can't keep up with demands of life.

(20+) Health Resource Burn Out: You are likely feeling completely overwhelmed and significant changes need to made in order to feel healthy and to meet the needs of daily living.

REFLECTIONS:

What is your definition of health? (Try to create a personal definition that is meaningful to you.)

_____

_____

In what are you mostly spending your health? (e.g., career, raising children, writing a book) Consider what you are spending your energy, abilities and time on. Is it worthy of you? Think about the four types of spending: Stress, Indulgent, Practical and Flow.

_____
_____
_____
_____
_____

What are you spending your health on that you feel is not worthwhile? Think about things you would like to do less. These may be in the areas of indulgent and stress spending.

_____
_____
_____
_____
_____

Where do you want to increase spending? What activities in either the areas of indulgent, practical or flow spending would you find rewarding, meaningful, pleasurable or practically useful?

_____
_____
_____
_____
_____

What are you doing (or could you be doing) to help heal, regenerate or improve your health? (e.g., spending time with friends, getting enough sleep, yoga, massage, going for regular walks outside, meditation, naps).

_____
_____
_____
_____
_____

ACTION

Consider your reflections from each area of health spending and health healing and write down **one** decision you have made to improve each area:

FLOW:

_____
_____
_____

PRACTICAL:

_____
_____
_____

INDULGENT:

_____
_____
_____

STRESS:

_____
_____
_____

ACTIVE HEALING:

_____
_____
_____

PASSIVE HEALING:

_____
_____
_____

Caring for one's health resource is a creative process that requires continual reflection, self-assessment, education and skill development. As we age, we need to update our approaches to adjust and adapt to the natural changes of the body in order to optimize health.

Being healthy is a creative process. The way each individual uses health resources or implements health healing in their life will vary based on their goals, personality, values, knowledge and experiences. Each health journey is unique for each individual. It takes work but the rewards make it worthwhile.

This journey is primarily about love: love of life, love of the body, love of movement, love of health. We focus on helping people and entire organizations connect to their health. Through the practice of movement, the mind and body come together and we can maintain a healthy connection throughout the day. We see the act of listening and meeting the needs of the body in any environment as an act of self-love.

Everyone has a unique reason for wanting to connect to their health. It might be to avoid sickness and pain, to enjoy life and have fun, or to be there for your family. Each person in the process of connecting to their health can discover their own motivations. What drives your desire for health?

9

Final Thoughts:
The Freedom to MOVE Forward

The vision of ThinkMOVE is to help people and organizations change the way they work and live so they can be healthy throughout the day. We do this primarily by helping people move away from the prison of chairs and desks to freely move their bodies. There are healthier and more productive ways to work that don't involve sitting 9.5 hours a day neglecting our bodies and destroying our health.

The ThinkMOVE program aims to create choices beyond established ways of working. We have engineered movement out of our lives for the sake of convenience and this has resulted in significant costs to our overall health and a separation between our minds and bodies. The choice and the freedom to MOVE in any context empowers people to be more flexible and adaptable both mentally and physically whether in relation to their career, relationships, or health. People who have more choices about their health and their bodies feel more in charge, autonomous, and powerful to live life to the fullest.

1. The Freedom of MOVEMENT Charter

Life appears to evolve constantly towards higher degrees of freedom. If you compare the mobility of any animal to humans, humans seem to have the most diverse array of movement possibilities. We are certainly the most free creature in terms of our ability to interact with and manipulate our environment and create tools (thank you, opposable thumbs!). We also have the greatest freedom of expression and communication through our voices and our ability to create complex languages.

Being sedentary is a side effect of our evolution towards more freedom. Thanks to technology, life has become easier and more convenient. Technologies like cars, cell phones, and the Internet have made transportation, communication, and information consumption more accessible, efficient, and less laborious. The side effect of all these benefits is the imprisonment of the body in chairs, cars, and couches, and behind desks and screens.

The ThinkMOVE program aims to help people free their bodies from the chains of their physical environments and any cultural assumptions that presuppose and/or limit what you can or cannot do with your own body in that environment.

For innovative companies, it's becoming clear that having people stuck to their chairs all day is not only detrimental to their health but to their productivity and the company's overall success. Empowering employees to have the freedom to move their bodies helps elevate the company to new levels of growth. The evidence is clear: Moving the body helps stimulate the mind so people are able to focus better and think more creatively about the challenges they face, in order to move beyond them.

I believe that Freedom to MOVE should become an integral part of every company's culture and formally in their health and safety policy. As discussed, the short- and long-term effects of being sedentary are significant whether they are from a financial, work productivity, or health perspective. Imagine the impact of a company entrusting and empowering employees to mind their bodies throughout the day: to move when their backs are feeling pain, when their bodies feel sore or stiff, or when they feel tired or mentally fatigued.

If the body is free then the mind is also free. Freeing the mind empowers innovative thinking which is the key to tomorrow's growth. In North America, we are afforded certain freedoms such as the freedom of thought, belief, opinion, and expression. We hope that one day everyone will be afforded the Freedom of Movement. Here are some preliminary ideas that companies and policy makers can use to support healthy movement at the workplace.

As an employee, I have the freedom to:

- Move my body whenever and however I would like as long as I am not interfering with someone else's rights or freedoms.

- Define how I work best for the needs and health of my body.

- Move and to make healthy choices and to not be judged or ridiculed for taking care of my health.

- Take time for my body periodically throughout the day as long as this does not interfere with my role and responsibilities to my employer.

As an employer, we aim to:

- Promote good physical and mental health education and practices in the workplace, and show a positive attitude to staff members who make efforts to care for their health.

- Create procedures and structures that support the health of staff and enable them to perform their jobs successfully while addressing the health issues related to prolonged sitting.

- Be a nonjudgmental leader through modeling and supporting staff to optimize their health through the Freedom to MOVE.

- Ensure all managers and supervisors have support and resources to encourage the Freedom to MOVE and address any health concerns relevant to the workplace.

In time, as the research on the negative impact of prolonged sitting increasingly enters into the public consciousness, people and companies will evolve in new ways, bringing new attitudes and policies that best account for the body's need for movement.

2. Moving towards Goals

As you embark on your journey and begin your own ThinkMOVE program, complete Exercise 17, which should help you get firm with your own goals.

3. Now It's Up to You

I feel that I have discovered the atoms and molecules of health and they are within the gift of movement. The possibilities and benefits of movement are as vast as the cosmos. I sincerely hope that you have found the information and the exercises in this book to be a helpful guide along your health journey. I truly believe that if we can learn to stay connected to our bodies and listen to its needs, whether at home or at work, there is a world of adventures waiting for us all.

Thank you for taking this journey with me and trusting me as your guide. Be well and MOVE well.

Exercise 17
Moving towards Goals Worksheet

Name: _____   **DATE:** _____

I'm so glad you've decided to take this step to improve your health and bring the power of movement into your everyday life.

This worksheet is where you will create your personal health destination. Taking the time to answer these questions will help you create an inspiring vision for your health so you'll know where you are going and why this is important for you.

Having clear goals will help you get the most out of the program. You will be able to leverage all the lessons, techniques, and practices so they move you towards *your* goals.

Try to complete this on your own. For some, it may be helpful to do this with someone whom you trust, who knows you well and who cares about you.

Try to be relaxed and centered in your body before you begin. Imagine, as honestly as you can, how you feel or how you would like to feel about what's being asked.

Try not to answer the questions from a purely logical perspective or what you think the "right" answers are. What's most important is what you want to experience.

It will take approximately **20** minutes to complete this. Take your time and don't rush this important step.

By doing this work you have already begun the change process since it demonstrates your commitment and effort. You will gain important insights that will help you understand what you want and what you will need to overcome any resistance to growth.

SECTION A: Where are you now? What's hurting?

You can think in terms of your physical, mental and relationship health. Be as honest as you can. No one else has to see your answers except you. You can use the <u>sentence stem</u> as a tool to help you generate answers. Repeat the suggested sentence stem five to ten times and answer spontaneously. Don't overthink. When you've completed five or ten stems you can review and elaborate on your answers.

1a.   What are your top three to five health complaints? Symptoms?

(Sentence Stem: "When it comes to my health, I am most concerned about...")

_____
_____
_____
_____

1b.   How are the things in #1 impacting your life currently? Think about how it impacts you in terms of your feelings, energy, self-perception.

(Sentence Stem: "Because of (answer from 1a), I notice/worry....")

_____
_____
_____
_____

2.   If you could resolve all that you listed in #1 what would be different about your life? What would change? Why is it important to address #1? How is problem X hindering your life (happiness, energy, vitality, work, relationships, self-confidence, mental health)?

(Sentence Stem: "If I didn't have (Answer to 1a), I would experience....")

_____
_____
_____
_____

3. Right now what is/are your biggest fears/worries concerning your health? Think long term whatever window of time that means for you. It could be two, five, 10, 25 years from now.

(Sentence Stem: "My biggest worry or fear in the long term is...")

_____
_____
_____
_____

3 b. How will your participation help with these fears/worries?

(Stem: "I hope I can...")

_____
_____
_____
_____

SECTION B: GOALS Creating an Exciting Future: Where would you like to go?

4a. If this program could help you change your current experience of your health, what would be different? What are the most important changes you are hoping to make regarding your health? Include as much detail as you can. Write something that's going to excite you and compel you to reach your goals.

Here is a stem to help you write out your vision:

Stem: "Seeing and experiencing myself reaching my ideal health a year from now, I am experiencing..."

(Consider your feelings, relationships and your work. Also, what changes would people notice about you from the outside?)

_____
_____
_____
_____
_____
_____

If more structure would help ...

Here is a list of some specific health areas you might consider. In addition to checking the boxes that apply to you, write out specific details below. Wherever possible be clear about how these changes will be observed or measured.

☐ What changes would you notice in terms of your energy? Increase energy, mental clarity (initiative, focus, productivity, etc.)

I will notice my energy: _____

☐ Weight loss — e.g., I would lose weight, feel more confident

I will lose _____ pounds and feel _____

☐ Productivity and focus:

I will notice: _____

☐ What differences would you notice in how you feel? Better mood? Feel happier? More positive outlook?

I will feel: _____

☐ What changes would you notice with your coworkers/team? Better team connection? Happier team?

With my colleagues I will notice: _____

☐ Pain: less stiffness, soreness, numbness and pain; more flexibility, mobility and ease (e.g., neck , back , shoulders, legs)

In my body I will notice: _____

☐ Increased job satisfaction

I will feel: _____

☐ Improved strength:

I will be able to: _____

☐ Improved cardio:

I will be able to: _____

☐ Improved flexibility:

I will be able to: _____

☐ Improved body awareness: awareness, posture, breathing:

I will notice: _____

☐ Improved self confidence or sense of attractiveness

I will see myself as: _____

☐ Improved balance/coordination:

I will be able to: _____

☐ Increased muscle tone:

I will notice: _____

☐ Improved appearance:

I will look: _____

☐ Improved stress management:

I will be able to: _____

Your ONE goal

Of everything that you wrote/selected above, pick the ONE goal that is most important to you that you hope to achieve.

My one and most important goal is to:

_____

Why is this ONE goal so important and why *must* you achieve this goal?

_____
_____
_____
_____

SECTION C: Strengths and Needs

What are your top three strengths? For example, open minded, hard working, creative, supportive, leadership, compassionate, intelligent, persistent.

1.

2.

3.

Think of **one way** you could you use these strengths to help you achieve your goals from Section B:

_____
_____
_____
_____
_____
_____
_____

Think of **one way** you could use your strengths to help others on your team:

_____
_____
_____
_____
_____
_____
_____

MY NEEDS:

In this section reflect on what challenges you will have on the way to achieving your goals.

- Consider things you have tried in the past. What worked well and why?
- What did not work well? Why did that not work well?
- What do **you** need to do (that worked well in the past) and /or do differently now so that you can be successful in this program?
- What do you need from **others** that will be helpful to your success?
- What will you need from **the program** to be successful?

As you reflect on the above questions, list in the table below what you will need from yourself, others, and the program. (We've listed some of the elements you'll be receiving from the program):

YOU ("To be successful, I need to ...")	OTHERS ("It would help me if others would ...") Colleagues, friends, family	Program ("What I need from the program is ...")
Example: Have a clear goal	Example: Invited/joined me on MOVE breaks	Tracking and accountability (Web application) Office-friendly movements Reminders/alerts through Web application Structure and a clear plan Others:

How comfortable are you right now with moving on your own at work throughout the day? Imagine doing stretches, strength, balance, cardio moves by your desk for a minute at a time. On a scale of one to five, five being the highest, how comfortable are you presently with moving on your own at work?

Not at all comfortable		Moderately comfortable		Very comfortable
1	2	3	4	5

What would help you to feel more comfortable (For example, time and practice, others joining you, manager's support and involvement)?

_____
_____
_____
_____
_____

Congrats! You are done. Keep this for your records. You'll reference this document several times through the six-week program. When you have completed the six-week program, review your answers here and reflect on how you have changed and whether you reached your goals.

Appendix:
Personal Health Declaration
and the Freedom to MOVE

The freedoms listed here form the foundation for the ThinkMOVE program. Each freedom represents important mindset shifts that will empower you and your team to move and be healthier throughout the day while addressing sedentary time.

In Part I, simply check off all the freedoms that fit for you and reflect how it would look and feel to actualize these freedoms in your daily life. In Part II, you'll write out your own Health Vision Statement based on the Moving towards Goals worksheet (Exercise 17).

These steps represent a commitment you make with yourself for your health. It is important to be clear about what change will look like and what it will take. There may be elements you would like to add that are not listed here. Please feel free to do so. If you notice concerns or barriers to any of the items below please consider receiving support from someone you trust or reaching out to the ThinkMOVE team (info@thinkmove.ca). We'd be happy to help.

Part I: Freedoms

I give myself the freedom and permission to:

- Prioritize my health and regard it as the foundation for all that I do and how I serve others.

- Be fully embodied which means to positively value and care for my entire body, not just my head.

- Move my body whenever, wherever, and however I would like and fits for me as long as I am not infringing on or interfering with someone else's rights or freedoms.

- Define for myself the ways I work and live best according to my needs and the health of my body.

- Live authentically and balancing my needs with others.

- Give and receive social support to and from those around me and create a social environment that supports positive health practices.

- Feel good about doing positive and nourishing things for myself daily.

- Move in all ways whether that is physically, mentally, or socially and to make healthy choices that fit for me and to not be judged or ridiculed for taking care of my health.

- Love my body with positive thoughts, appreciations and actions and let go of judgments or feelings of guilt or shame (my own or others) that may attempt to interfere with me taking care of my health.

- Take time for my body periodically with regular movement breaks throughout the day as long as this does not interfere with my roles and responsibilities.

- Learn and grow which means that sometimes I will make mistakes and not always get things right. I don't expect myself to be perfect, but simply to grow in my abilities day by day and to keep trying and practicing.

- Have fun and enjoy my body, which means using myself playfully and creatively. It also means celebrating my efforts and achievements and others.

- Other: _____

- Other: _____

Part II: Vision

My Personal Health Vision Statement

(Reference your Moving towards Goals worksheet (Exercise 17), particularly sections A and B).

I am committed to incorporating health practices into my day so I can experience:

_____

_____

_____

_____

… and I can avoid (reference your section A):

_____

_____

_____

_____

… and in the long run I can (reference section B):

_____

_____

_____

_____

ThinkMOVE participant:

Name: _____

Signature: _____

Date: _____

Witness: _____

Download Kit

Please enter the URL you see in the box below in a web browser on your computer to access and use the download kit.

www.self-counsel.com/updates/moveordie/17kit.htm

The following files are included in the download kit:

- Written exercises to get you thinking about moving
- A ThinkMOVE journal you can use to track your progress
- Web resources, further readings, and more!